PRAISE FOR
What's Stressing Your Face?

"Dr. Ablon's book is brilliant. The stories are relatable and engage the reader at every step. She clarifies the mind and skin connection, validates holistic approaches, and offers a range of valuable treatments. This book is going to be a big hit! No reader will want to put it down."

—Doris Day, M.D., F.A.A.D., Clinical Associate Professor, Dermatology, NYU Langone Medical Center, New York, N.Y.

"This book is an excellent resource for both doctors and patients. Dr Ablon brings in hard science, with real data, and breaks it down so it's usable. She has discussed novel treatment techniques that I will certainly consider adding in my own practice."

—Andrew P. Ordon, M.D., F.A.C.S.,
Host, the Emmy Award-winning The Doctors, TV

"Dr. Ablon goes into detail about how [illegible] ıct many skin disorders. She [illegible] solutions you can i[illegible]

—Howard Mur[illegible]
Associate Clinic[illegible]

What's Stressing Your Face?

A DOCTOR'S GUIDE TO PROACTIVE AGING AND HEALING: ROSACEA, HAIR LOSS, PSORIASIS, SHINGLES AND OTHER FACIAL CONDITIONS

GLYNIS ABLON, M.D., F.A.A.D.
with Susanna DeSimone, M.F.A.

Dear Lissy,
Not like you have any stress in your life... live your best stress-less life!
♥ G

Basic Health
PUBLICATIONS, INC.

The information contained in this book is based upon the research and personal and professional experiences of the authors. It is not intended as a substitute for consulting with your physician or other healthcare provider. Any attempt to diagnose and treat an illness should be done under the direction of a healthcare professional.

The publisher does not advocate the use of any particular healthcare protocol but believes the information in this book should be available to the public. The publisher and authors are not responsible for any adverse effects or consequences resulting from the use of the suggestions, preparations, or procedures discussed in this book. Should the reader have any questions concerning the appropriateness of any procedures or preparation mentioned, the authors and the publisher strongly suggest consulting a professional healthcare advisor.

Basic Health Publications, Inc.
885 Claycraft Road
Columbus, OH 43230
800.334.9969 • www.basichealthpub.com

Library of Congress Cataloging-in-Publication Data is available through the Library of Congress.

Editor: Roberta W. Waddell
Typesetting/Book design: Gary A. Rosenberg
Cover design: Kimberly Richey

Printed in the United States of America

10 9 8 7 6 5 4 3 2 1

Contents

Part Three—Innovative Treatments

Part Four—Non-Invasive Skin Treatments and Procedures

Acknowledgments

When I took on the challenge of writing this book, it impacted those around me—from my family, to co-workers, friends, and even my patients. It is thanks to these people that I have written this book. My thanks go to the thousands of patients who have told me their stories (names have been changed in some cases to protect identities), listened to my advice, and implemented my suggestions in their daily lives. Thanks also go to my family for their advice, love, and support, to my staff at Ablon Skin Institute and Research Center, to Norman Goldfind and Basic Health Publications for supporting the message of my book, to my editor Bobby Waddell for her exceptional work on this project, and to my friends who have cared and understood my crazed upheaval and distraction while writing this. I could name names, but you know who you are, and from the bottom of my heart, I say thank you, thank you, thank you. May this book help you find the peace, harmony, balance, and happiness we all deserve. May it help you reduce stress and see the world for the beauty and wonders it holds. May you experience every day for the gift it is, find balance, and realize, as I have, that stress only wastes, damages, and destroys the precious moments of your life.

Introduction

"There's a chance your facial paralysis could be permanent." The doctor's words echoed in my head, inciting an array of fears. *Will my kids be frightened by my looks?* I couldn't move the left side of my face. Half of my mouth drooped oddly, and one eyebrow sloped downward. As a dermatologist and cosmetic surgeon, Bell's palsy was an ironic affliction to be stricken by. *How could I assert myself as a facial doctor if I couldn't move one side of my face?* I couldn't help but wonder, *Will my patients trust my medical expertise? Why has this happened to me?*

As I examined my life over that year, I realized my health crisis was due to the horrendous amount of stress I had been under. I thought I was handling the stress because I was still functioning. Clearly, I wasn't—because *it* was now handling me. Over time, it had accumulated in my body and worn down my immune system. Oblivious as I was to its toll on my health, it took this startling crisis to get my attention in a way that would cause me to seek change.

I am not alone in experiencing a stress-induced facial condition. Throughout my eighteen years of practicing medicine as a dermatologist and cosmetic surgeon, I have consistently witnessed one prevailing issue among my patients—stress. Their steady stream of similar stories demonstrates this alarming trend. Take, for example,

Shana, a litigator whose stress mounted with her excruciating hours and harried court cases until her hair began to fall out. Then there was Alice, a single mother, who plodded through exhausting work weeks while trying to balance the needs of her toddler until a painful rash erupted on her face. Or Chad, a small business owner, who struggled to care for his ailing daughter and manage the demands of his office, until his scalp psoriasis skyrocketed out of control. What all these stories have in common, including my own, is that acute stress was wreaking havoc on the skin.

For most people, the road to a stress-induced facial ailment does not happen overnight. Instead, it is a long trek where the stress slowly and silently erodes your health until one day you look in the mirror and notice sudden aging or hair loss, or an outbreak of rosacea, or an eruption of psoriasis. Often, it is not until these noticeable types of physical symptoms affect your face that you begin to heed the stress you are under. In my case, my stress-induced facial palsy occurred after the most taxing nine months of my life, even though I thought I had everything under control.

The entire nightmare began in the unlikeliest of places—on vacation. The Palm Desert sun warmed my body as I relaxed by the pool, shielded under an umbrella, and slathered in water-resistant/zinc-based sunscreen with a sun-protection factor of 50. This was the family getaway that I looked forward to all year. I called up to my mother to come join me by the pool. She didn't answer. I became concerned because she hadn't been feeling well that day, which she attributed to having a tad too much to drink at the previous night's dinner. I padded into our hotel room where, to my horror, I discovered her sprawled on the bed and unresponsive to my cries. My father and I rushed her to a nearby hospital where she was diagnosed with bacterial meningitis.

This traumatic event kicked off nine months of consecutive health catastrophes for my mother. Against all odds, she managed to recover from one illness, only to have another huge setback in her health—while recovering from the meningitis, the meningitis-specific medicine caused a bowel perforation. After she recovered from the perforated bowel, she developed aspiration pneumonia. During this entire period, I struggled to balance my time and energies between tending to my ailing mother, meeting the high-pressure demands of running my medical practice, and attending to the daily needs of my young children. I was stretched to the max in many different directions, and realized I was experiencing a lot of stress (or *duress,* as constant stress is referred to). Yet, I reasoned that, since I was handling everything, it must not be getting to me. Little did I know, however, that my stress was slowly destroying my health.

One morning when I awoke, I knew something was drastically wrong. At first, I couldn't place it. A tingling sound echoed deep in my ears, and my face felt numb. When I saw my reflection in the mirror, I gasped. The left side of my face drooped oddly. I tried to smile, but discovered I couldn't move the left side of my mouth. Upon further self-examination, I found I could barely move my forehead (this is actually a good sign, because with a stroke I would have been able to move my forehead). Based on my symptoms, I deduced that I was suffering from an onslaught of Bell's palsy. While dialing my physician, I took the first-line medications used to treat Bell's palsy—steroids and a high dose of Acyclovir. During the appointment with my physician, the diagnosis was confirmed—I, indeed, had Bell's palsy.

My story, and the stories of my patients who have experienced facial ailments due to stress, all share a common thread—living with extreme stress had become the norm. Our relationship with stress was akin to a hissing scorpion in a corner that we ignored, perhaps under the cover of coping. So, having ignored the presence of the scorpion, which should have elicited terror and a decisive removal action, the menacing threats were tolerated until a strike left each of us aghast at the frightening results on our faces. This is exactly what long-term stress does to you. It rises up quietly until it strikes you in some visible and/or painful way you can't ignore.

These types of experiences are widespread. As these studies show, stress is affecting the health of our nation.

- 43 percent of all adults experience adverse health effects from stress.[1]
- 75–90 percent of all doctor's office visits are for stress-related ailments and complaints.[2]
- The Occupational Safety and Health Administration (OSHA) declared stress a hazard of the workplace. Stress costs American industry more than $300 billion annually.[3]

Studies also reveal that stress deteriorates the health of the face and hair in some of the following ways:

- Aging. "Researchers estimated that each tiny increase in a key stress hormone, cortisol… aged a person by about half a year."[4]
- Hair thinning. While genetics play a part in this, stress is also a key factor. "A 2012 study of 98 pairs of identical female twins found that the sisters who reported the most stress in their lives also had the most hair loss.[5]
- Rosacea outbreaks. "More than 16 million Americans suffer from rosacea." A National Rosacea Society survey shows that stress is a triggering factor in 79 percent of cases.[6]
- Psoriasis outbreaks. "As many as 7.5 million Americans suffer from psoriasis.[7] Studies have found that the proportion of stress-induced psoriasis cases ranges from 37–78 percent.[8]

As these statistics showcase, stress can have a dramatic impact on your appearance, especially your face, skin, and hair. Your skin is intimately connected to the functioning of your organs and your hormonal changes. Stress can upset your internal balance and release an influx of hormones, such as cortisol, testosterone, and dehydroepiandrosterone (DHEA). Stress also decreases the production of estrogen, progesterone, melatonin, growth hormones, and thyroid hormones. Over time, the harmful effects of these hormonal changes show up on your face, skin, and hair. These effects can range from a minor rash to a life-changing malady, such as paralysis.

For these reasons, I knew that my path to healing had to involve more than treating my facial symptoms. It had to involve taking charge of my stress. In my own journey to healing my Bell's palsy, I utilized the same trifecta of treatments that I prescribe to my patients who have a stress-induced facial condition.

- Holistic treatments
- Cutting-edge technological treatments; and
- Non-invasive skin treatments

Through these treatments and techniques, I was able to take control of my stress, and recover complete control of my facial muscles, expression, and function.

For years, my patients have requested that I write a book detailing my methods for creating and maintaining beautiful skin. I felt that such a book must address the ill effects of stress, as well. As a result, I've written this book to help the many readers who are living with the effects of stress on their face, skin, and hair, and are unsure what to do about it. Whether those effects are in the form of rosacea, premature aging, hair loss, or migraines, I want to share with you the path to healing that has worked for my patients and for me. This book takes you into my office where you are made privy to the same medical insights into stress-induced facial ailments that I provide for my patients. In the following pages, as today's proven treatments and techniques are explored, you will find hope for healing your stress-induced face, skin, and/or hair condition.

The material is divided into four sections. The first section, Chapters 1–4, presents real-life stories of my patients to demonstrate how stress affects the face from the inside out. Each chapter in this section will examine a stress-related struggle concerning skin ailments, aging, hair conditions, or nerve issues. At the end of each chapter's discussion of a stress-induced facial issue, treatment options will be provided, and the relevant chapters on that specific treatment will be referenced. This will allow you to locate the sections that best apply to you within Chapters 5–14, where in-depth explanations of therapeutic techniques are provided.

It is my goal that through reading my book you will be able to reclaim the health of your face from the ravages of stress. This means you will have learned to not only treat the physical symptoms of your skin condition, but to also address the root cause of these symptoms—your stress. Through doing this, you will not only heal your skin, but live a better, healthier life.

UPDATE

It's been more than two years since the start of the troubles for us. My mom has survived more challenges and lives life to its fullest everyday–she is my hero. My dad is by her side every step of the way.

My Bell's Palsy has for the most part been resolved; the stabbing pain in my ear and jaw is gone, but I continue to have dryness and eye irritation on the affected side of my face. With eye drops, reading glasses, and rest, I easily negotiate these minor issues. So, no complaints.

I wake up each day now and enjoy my daily existence–from my family, to my work, to my play. Now, I truly feel I have found, not just the balance, but also the peace and harmony I never thought I could have in my life. I teach my children to live and love and cherish every moment, every event, every hope and dream. I tell my patients every day to live life to the fullest. Life is short.

PART ONE

Stress-Related Facial Problems

SKIN CONDITIONS

Chapter 1 uses the experiences of my patients to explore the link between stress and skin conditions, such as rashes, psoriasis, rosacea, eczema, and shingles. Therapeutic options for healing are discussed, and you are referred to the corresponding chapters that examine each type of therapy in detail.

AGING

Chapter 2 discusses the aging process, and draws on my patients' experiences to explore how stress can speed up this process and incite worry wrinkles, sunspots, and thinning skin. This chapter also discusses the influx of stress hormones that ensue during menopause, and the rapid aging that occurs as a result. An overview of treatment options is provided, and you are referred to the corresponding chapters that discuss each treatment in further detail.

HAIR CONDITIONS

Chapter 3 examines the link between stress and hair conditions, including hair loss, unwanted hair growth, and the hormonal changes that occur during menopause. Each section includes a real-life scenario of one of my patients to illustrate the link between stress and their hair condition, and provides treatment options with references to the chapters that explore each type of healing therapy in more detail.

NERVE CONDITIONS

Chapter 4 dissects how stress can trigger nerve-related conditions. This chapter uses my patients' experiences with stress-induced migraines, and my experience with stress-induced Bell's palsy, to examine the association between stress and these conditions. Therapeutic options to heal these conditions are discussed, and you are referred to the chapters that focus on these specific treatments.

It is my goal that, through reading my book, you will be able to reclaim the health of your face from the ravages of stress. This means you will have learned to both treat the physical symptoms of your skin condition and address the root cause of these symptoms—your stress. Through doing this, you will not only heal your skin, but will live a better, healthier life going forward.

1

Stress and Skin

Skin Overview

Your skin is a reflection of your internal being.

It is well known that the eyes are a window to your soul, but it is not widely known that the skin is, similarly, a window to your emotional state. Your skin reflects your internal life, especially when you are under stress. The largest organ of your body, your skin, is comprised of nerves, blood vessels, hair follicles, oil and sweat glands, as well as connective tissue, muscle, and fat. There are two main layers in your skin, the inner layer, known as the dermis, and the outer layer, known as the epidermis.

Your skin organ receives information from the outer world and from inner hormonal processes. This is why your skin responds to external changes, such as temperature, and responds to such internal changes as an influx of hormones caused by stress. Although a little stress can be helpful in getting your body revved up and ready to go, chronic stress can do just the opposite. In times of stress, or *dis*tress, as chronic stress has been labeled, cortisol (known as the stress hormone) and other hormones increase, including glucocorticoids and adrenal androgens that cause the sebaceous gland to overproduce an oily substance. This gland, which is connected to your hair follicles, releases its oily substance through the pores of your skin, and when too much of it is released onto your skin, it can trigger acne, rashes, and rosacea. An influx of stress hormones also causes your skin to become more susceptible to inflammation, and can incite, or worsen, flare-ups of rashes, psoriasis, rosacea, eczema, and shingles. The following chapters chronicle personal stories of my patients to illustrate the link between stress and these conditions, and provide a combination of Eastern and Western medical treatment options.

Sabrina's Embarrassment About Her Rashes

During her morning ritual, Sabrina, a fifty-four-year old Middle-Eastern woman, scrubbed her face with fierce intensity in a hopeless attempt to ward off the raised pink spots that dotted her forehead. She knew they were the telltale signs that a rash was coming on, and knew that, as the morning progressed, she could expect the bumps to spread into a circular red lesion on her forehead. With mounting anxiety, she imagined how the afternoon managerial meeting at her office would go as her co-workers tried not to stare at the swollen red sores protruding on her face. Michelle, her coworker, would bury her head in the report and avoid looking at Sabrina. Steve would speak to Sabrina slowly, enunciating each word as if her facial condition impaired her hearing. Others would look on sympathetically, while they wondered what was wrong with Sabrina's face.

The truth is that Sabrina wondered the same thing. Despite all the treatments she had sought out, this rash had sporadically plagued her for the last fifteen years. The humiliation of the whole thing made Sabrina want desperately to call in sick, but she had already missed too much work because she had used up all her sick time handling the many diverse arrangements connected to the recent passing of her mother.

To make matters worse, on top of dealing with the loss of her mom, her best friend and the grounding force in her family, a bitter battle over the division of her mother's estate broke out between Sabrina and her siblings. It was heart-wrenching and exhausting for Sabrina to cope with the feuding, which turned what was once a tight-knit family into a tattered mess.

Meanwhile, Sabrina's rash kept erupting on her face. Fed up after fifteen years of this, Sabrina came to see me. By that time, her rash had come and gone many times, for inexplicable reasons. My search for the source of this rash involved more than seven biopsies, more than one laboratory blood workup, and x-rays. All diagnoses pointed toward *figurate erythema,* a rash that tends to erupt in circular red lesions. I prescribed oral steroids, and Sabrina's rash did clear up for a while, but soon she was back in my office.

As Sabrina and I discussed her current life situation, it became clear that her mother's death, and the subsequent war over the inheritance with her siblings, was quite possibly the source of the emotional stress that kept triggering her outbreaks. Since her rash had a tendency to erupt after emotionally taxing moments, it was clear that I needed to address the root cause of Sabrina's rash instead of falling back on the traditional treatment of oral steroids, which was only addressing her symptoms.

In the end, and after three weeks of effectively employing the stress-management exercises and therapies I prescribed, ninety percent of her rash had cleared up.

Dr. Ablon's Medical Analysis of Rashes, Such as Sabrina's

> After long-term stress has weakened the immune system, outbreaks of stress-induced rashes can occur.

Oftentimes when there is a recurring rash, the problem appears to be the condition itself, but, in actuality, the problem is unregulated stress. While studies have yet to find the exact mechanism that causes stress-induced rashes, it is known that outbreaks occur after long-term stress has weakened the immune system. A rash on the skin indicates that the skin has succumbed to some irritation or inflammation. Under normal circumstances, the skin acts as a barrier to irritants with the help of the immune system. When the immune system has been impaired by stress, however, the skin's ability to act as a barrier is diminished. This occurs because the immune system is specifically made to function under short-term, not long-term stress. In fact, short-term stress can be a good thing—it can provide a boost and help the body fight off an infection. Ongoing stress, however, has the opposite effect on the immune system, depressing it and making the skin more susceptible to irritation that can trigger, or worsen, such skin conditions as rashes.[1]

Many people with chronic stress experience a stress-related breakout on their skin. My patients who have experienced recurring rashes due to emotional stress found that their symptoms did not clear up with conventional treatments. In their cases, stress-management techniques, in addition to other treatments, were needed to address their condition.

Stress-induced rashes can take on a variety of visible forms, such as raised red bumps, hives, or welts, or they may appear as circular red patches, just to name a few. A recurring rash can also be a symptom of a chronic skin condition, such as psoriasis, rosacea, or eczema, which is triggered, or made worse, by stress. Psoriasis generally appears in plaques on the skin, which look like raised, red, inflamed lesions covered by dry scaly skin, and typically break out on the scalp, knees, elbows, fold of buttocks, and penile shaft. Rosacea, another chronic condition, often appears as patches of redness or flushing on the nose, cheeks, forehead, and chin. For some people, the symptoms of rosacea appear as bumps, lesions, or pimples, which look similar to acne. Eczema usually consists of tiny blisters on red, swollen patches of skin. Sometimes the blisters erupt and a thin crust forms over the inflamed skin.

It is important to seek the advice of a dermatologist in order determine the cause of your rash. A dermatologist will analyze the identifying characteristics of your rash in order ascertain the source of your skin's irritation, and may also take a sample of the skin for microscopic inspection. Identifying factors include the location of the rash on the body, color, shape, and size of inflamed skin.

In order to figure out if your rash is stress-induced, it is important to rule out other possible causes, including allergic reactions to foods or external contact with an irritating substance, such as a plant or a product (soap, shampoo). Other common causes of rashes include fungal or yeast infections of the skin, both of which can be treated by antifungal creams. Rashes can also be symptomatic of a bacterial infection in the skin that needs to be treated by antibiotics. If the cause of your rash cannot be attributed to factors other than your stress, then it is referred to as a *non-specific rash,* and is more than likely stress-induced.

Treatment Options for Rashes, Such as Sabrina's

> If you are suffering from a rash during or after an emotionally trying time, stress-management techniques are an important part of your healing plan.

To treat stress-induced rashes, I recommend a multifaceted holistic approach, which combines meditation, massage, breathing, and movement exercises, plus acupuncture, nutrition, and supplements, in conjunction with skin treatments, such as light-emitting diode therapy, pulsed electromagnetic therapy, floating therapy, and anti-inflammatory creams.

If you are experiencing a rash during or after an emotionally trying time, stress-management techniques are an important part of your healing plan. This includes adding relaxation exercises—meditation, massage, floating therapy, or breathing, and such movement work as yoga—to your weekly schedule. These practices serve to regulate your breathing, heart rate, and metabolism. As a result, they reduce the physical and emotional consequences of stress, and create a sense of well-being, which, in turn, reduces stress hormones, thus decreasing the activation of inflammation in the skin.

How Miguel Was Helped by These Treatments

Miguel, a fifty-four-year-old Hispanic man, came to me after undergoing chemotherapy for intestinal cancer, and had a type of rash known as an *erythematous papular rash* all over his face. At first, thinking it could be a reaction to the chemotherapy, I prescribed a round of topical anti-inflammatory medication. But he was soon back in my office, as the medication had not abated his rash and the next step was to delve into how his fight with cancer was affecting his life and his family. "It's terribly stressful," he admitted.

I recommended that he incorporate meditation, yoga, and floating therapy into his schedule once a week. I also suggested that he reduce his intake of high glycemic-index foods that trigger inflammation, and begin to incorporate supplements into his regular routine. Additionally, he began light-emitting diode therapy and pulsed electromagnetic therapy for his skin. Within six weeks, Miguel relayed to me that he had a better sense of well-being, and his rash had completely cleared up.

Nutritional supplements are beneficial in boosting the immune system to help prevent the outbreak of stress-induced rashes. Vitamin C is particularly helpful because it is the primary vitamin needed for the production of collagen, a structural protein in skin, and is a necessary nutrient involved in the process of transmitting nerve impulses and hormones. Vitamin B-complex helps to support the immune system, and Vitamin E, an antioxidant, works to protect against cell-membrane damage and, as studies have shown, is an important support for the immune system. There are also a variety of minerals that are beneficial in supporting it as well.

When treating stress-induced rashes, light-emitting diode therapy is also beneficial because it uses bursts of light energy to decrease inflammation and break down damaged skin cells so healthy cells can grow.

Topical anti-inflammatory creams and barrier-repair creams can also help to heal stress-induced rashes. These function to reduce swelling and prevent the occurrence of more skin inflammation by forming a protective layer of skin cells. Pyratine cream and brimonidine gels are also useful for treating stress-induced rashes.

When dealing with stressful life situations, psychotherapy is a helpful treatment that can serve to alleviate stress and clear up ensuing stress-related skin conditions.

For those who are experiencing stress-related rashes, the above therapies can clear up the irritated skin and prevent recurrences.

Psoriasis

Chad's Embarrassment with Psoriasis

Chad, a thirty-four year old Hispanic male, held the hand of his three-year-old daughter, Lily, as she wiggled under the nurse's touch. The nurse, a young brunette who looked like she was straight out of college, deftly went about the job of inserting an IV into his daughter's arm. Chad tried to relax as he caressed Lily's matted hair, but as he stared at her pale face, fears marched through his head. *What if my daughter never recovers from her kidney infection? Will she have a normal life?* When the nurse finished with the IV, she turned her gaze toward Chad. He could feel her scrutiny and knew instantly that she was assessing his condition. "How long have you had that?" she asked gently. Chad squirmed, embarrassed.

The nurse drew closer to Chad, examining the silvery, scaled patches of raised skin all over his neck and scalp. Chad had struggled with psoriasis for years, but since Lily had been in the hospital, it had mushroomed out of control. Red, scaly patches spread from his scalp, down his neck and back, then crept along his legs until they covered 80 percent of his body. Whenever Chad left the house, it was a struggle to hide his condition. And having to don his hooded sweatshirt every time he went out in public made him feel like a leper. It was especially difficult to cover up adequately at work, since he was required to wear a suit, leaving his neck and scalp precariously exposed.

The nurse waited for Chad's response. He shrugged. "I have creams for it," he said. "Are they working?" she queried.

This question reverberated in Chad's head. Since Lily had been in the hospital, his creams had not made a dent in the itchy, sore, flaky patches. He was in constant pain, but was so absorbed with his daughter's condition that he didn't know where to start with his own.

The topical creams had stopped working for Chad. His case, in fact, illustrated a clear connection between the worsening of his condition and the trauma of dealing with his daughter's severe illness.

Chad conveyed that he constantly struggled to hide his outbreaks. How could he go to work and interact with his co-workers and clients when he had red splotches all over his scalp and neck, along with dandruff-like scales that were continually shedding onto the collar and shoulders of his dark suits?

After visiting me and using my recommended treatments–meditation, light-emitting diode therapy, dietary changes, supplements, floating-tank therapy, exercise, acupuncture, and prescription creams–Chad saw a huge improvement in his condition within two months.

Dr. Ablon's Medical Analysis of Psoriasis Conditions, Such as Chad's

> The connection between psoriasis and stress can be linked to the chemicals in your brain.

Psoriasis is a chronic autoimmune disease of the skin. It affects "upwards of 7.5 million Americans," and is "the most common autoimmune disease in the country," according to the National Psoriasis Foundation.[2] In autoimmune diseases, the immune system turns on itself and attacks a good substance that is supposed to be in the body, such as our tissue, instead of the bad substance that is not supposed to be in our body, such as an infection. There are several types of psoriasis. The most common type, plaque psoriasis, looks like raised, red, inflamed lesions covered by dry scaly skin. These lesions are painful, itchy, flaky, and uncomfortable for those who are beset by them.

Psoriasis is a complex disease with several factors involved in the onset of this skin condition. Both a genetic predisposition and defects in the immune system play a part in developing this disease. On a cellular level, psoriasis can be attributed to a problem with the turnover of cells in the most common type of skin cell—keratinocytes. These cells function to make the protein keratin, which serves to strengthen the skin, hair, and nails. When there is a defect in these cells, it results in a rapid increase in the replacement of new cells. This causes so many new cells to be created that it leads to the formation of the classic silvery-scaled plaques, typically found on the scalp, knees, elbows, fold of the buttocks, and penile shaft.

The involvement of the immune system is multifaceted as there are several deficiencies in it that can incite psoriasis. Recent research has demonstrated that psoriatic patches may occur when the immune system mistakenly recognizes healthy cells as abnormal. This activates proteins called *inflammasomes,* and they send signals to neurochemical pathways to trigger the skin inflammation associated with psoriasis. Psoriasis can also be attributed to a defect in the turnover of a cell-surface molecule that mediates the interactions of the immune system (known as the human leucocyte antigen system). This molecule is involved in the process of fighting off infections, and determines how susceptible a person is to an autoimmune disease.

Environmental factors, such as stress, play a big role in the onset of psoriasis, as well. In fact, many people do not know they are prone to psoriasis until they go through a stressful time in their life and develop this condition. The majority of those who develop psoriasis come to consider that stress is "the main cause for exacerbation of their psoriasis." While there are other trigger factors, such as cold temperatures, alcohol, infection (especially respiratory), hypertension, diet (especially foods high in carbohydrates that can spike blood-sugar levels), most people rank stress as the primary culprit in their outbreaks.[3] These findings are consistently verified by studies, which "support a relationship between stress and psoriasis."[4]

The connection between psoriasis and stress can be linked to brain chemicals because, during times of stress, chemical neurotransmitters are released from the brain. This surge of brain chemicals weakens the immune system, increases skin inflammation, and diminishes the skin's ability to act as a barrier against irritants. This lessening of the barrier allows for an increase in skin permeability and the subsequent outbreaks of the scaly coating and red lesions attributed to psoriasis. Now, there are new biologic drugs available, which serve to target the hormones that induce skin inflammation.[5]

Every time there is an outbreak (and aside from its physical component), psoriasis psychologically torments those affected with a range of negative emotions, especially if the diseased skin is visible. In the case of visible red sores or patches of white scales, people often feel embarrassed and humiliated. Studies have confirmed that those who develop this condition due to stress find it more emotionally traumatizing than those whose psoriasis is not stress-related. According to one study, those who experienced stress-induced psoriasis tended to not only have more "plaques of psoriasis on visible areas," but also to "self-report a greater disease severity than" those whose psoriasis was not stress-induced.[5]

This often results in a vicious cycle where people who have stress-induced psoriasis experience an onslaught of this condition after a stressful time in their life; then the outbreak causes more emotional stress, which, in turn, worsens their psoriasis, thus making their condition less likely to respond to treatment.

Treatment Options for Psoriasis Conditions, Such as Chad's

> Decreasing stress can reduce the severity of a psoriasis outbreak, and help prevent recurrences.

If you are aggravated by stress-induced psoriasis, reducing stress is paramount. Decreasing stress can reduce the severity of the outbreak, as well as help to prevent recurrences. Therefore, you need a therapeutic approach that not only treats your symptoms, but also addresses your stress.

For anyone with stress-related psoriasis, the first major change I recommend is incorporating a holistic treatment, such as getting a massage, or practicing meditation or yoga, on a weekly basis. For more details on how to implement meditation, relaxation, and movement techniques to treat your skin condition, please refer to Chapters 5 and 7. For details on how massage functions as a stress reducer, and the different types of massage therapy, please refer to Chapter 6.

Acupuncture is an excellent holistic option to treat stress-induced psoriasis as it has the ability to decrease heart rate and blood pressure, and relax muscles, which can, in turn, reduce stress. Eastern medicine holds that stress blocks the flow of energy. Acupuncture corrects the flow of energy, and this acts to minimize stress and the symptoms of stress. Please refer to Chapter 8 for a full discussion of the history and philosophy of acupuncture.

When dealing with stressful life situations, psychotherapy is a useful treatment that can alleviate stress and clear up consequent stress-related skin conditions. For a discussion of the benefits of this therapy and the techniques or approaches available, turn to Chapter 10.

Another treatment that is useful in healing inflammation and clearing up skin plaques is light-emitting diode therapy. In fact, a study I conducted at the Ablon Skin Institute and Research Center with chronic psoriasis patients found that light-emitting diode therapy is a particularly effective treatment option for persistent cases that have not responded to topical medication alone and other conventional treatments.[6] For further discussion on how light-emitting diode therapy functions to heal psoriasis plaques, please refer to Chapter 11.

People with psoriasis can also apply prescription creams to reduce inflammation. Studies show that vitamin-D topical cream inhibits the inflammatory reaction that initiates psoriasis. Topical steroid creams are also helpful because they function as anti-inflammatories that work to reduce the swelling and inflammation of psoriatic lesions. Tazarotene is a topical vitamin-A derivative that causes the thinning of psoriatic plaques and allows all other therapies to work better. For more details on prescription creams, turn to Chapter 13.

Food also plays a role in psoriasis outbreaks. Limiting the consumption of foods that trigger inflammation, such as eggs, fatty meat, fried foods, alcohol, and processed sugar, can be an important preventive measure. I recommend following the guidelines of the book, *Win the War Within: The Eating Plan That's Clinically Proven to Fight Inflammation—The Hidden Cause of Weight Gain and Chronic Disease*, by Dr. Floyd Chilton. For specific nutritional guidelines on this type of low inflammatory diet, please refer to Chapter 9.

There are many helpful supplements that serve to reduce plaque formation on the skin, including milk thistle, which inhibits inflammatory compounds, and omega-3 fatty acids, which reduce inflammation of the skin. Other vitamins and minerals that can help create the formation of healthy skin include vitamin C, vitamin B-complex, vitamin B_{12}, vitamin E, calcium, magnesium, and beta-carotene. For more details on their healing capabilities and the positive effects each of these supplements has on the body, please turn to Chapter 9.

The Healing Benefits of Multiple Treatment Methods for Psoriasis

If you are experiencing stress-induced psoriasis, a combination of holistic methods and cutting-edge prescription creams and treatments can work together to heal symptoms and control outbreaks—although recalcitrant psoriasis conditions may need more extensive treatment. One of my patients, Elizabeth, a sixty-three-year-old Caucasian attorney, had one such case. Her psoriasis included plaque formations and was so severe that, prior to seeing me, she had been on a medication generally prescribed for oral cancer that is known for its possible harmful effects on the liver. She had also undergone a type of ultraviolet light therapy, which had disastrously left her with multiple sites of skin cancer. As we discussed her lifestyle and the stressors in her life, it became clear that her work as a litigator was extremely taxing emotionally. She could not reduce her hours at work, so I suggested she begin a five-minute meditation period twice a day—once prior to work, and a second time before heading home. She did incorporate this into her daily routine, and in addition got a massage every two weeks and had floating-tank sessions once a month. We made changes to her diet, added specific supplements to her daily routine, and got her started using topical vitamin-D cream and tazarotene cream, also incorporating light-emitting diode therapy into her regimen. After following up on my recommended range of treatments, her condition was greatly improved. These combined treatments worked together to rapidly diminish her plaque formations and she is happy to report that all her psoriasis symptoms are now under control.

Rosacea

Fred's Trepidation

It was the morning of Fred's daughter's wedding. In the months leading up to this day, Fred, a sixty-one-year-old male Caucasian, assumed it would be a joyous morning filled with anticipation. What he did not expect, however, was to look in the mirror and find large red patches of acne all over his face. Instead of being excited, he was filled with dread at the thought of having to face the wedding guests. This type of predicament is more common for a kid in high school than for a man in his sixties, he thought.

Fred and his daughter, Brie, were very close. When she came to him with the news of her engagement, Fred wanted to give her the wedding of her dreams. This desire became complicated by the immense size of her fiancé's family and the need to include all their extended relatives. Securing a location big enough to fit their combined families took on a life of its own, and as a result, the price of the wedding soared while Fred's bank account dwindled. Throughout the whole process, Fred continued to smile because he didn't want to show how stressed he felt, and he wanted his daughter to have a beautiful celebration. As the big day neared, red sores erupted all over his face. At first he thought it was acne, and tried over-the-counter products to relieve it, but that only made it worse. Fred remembered feeling embarrassed at the rehearsal dinner. He gave a speech to their joint families, but instead of feeling he could hold his head high, he was terribly self-conscious about the pimples all over his face. In spite of this, the wedding he gave his daughter was a great success, but afterwards Fred knew he needed to seek help, and this is when he came to see me. Once Fred incorporated the holistic techniques I recommended for dealing with his stress, in addition to the other skin treatments I administered, his outbreaks of rosacea dissipated, to his great relief.

Dr. Ablon's Medical Analysis of Rosacea Conditions, Such as Fred's

Stress is a triggering factor in 79 percent of rosacea cases.[7]

Rosacea is a chronic skin disease that strikes in the adult years of thirty and beyond, and tends to affect fair-skinned individuals. A sudden outbreak in adulthood can be really traumatizing for anyone who never had to struggle with acne in adolescence. Known as *erythematotelangiectatic rosacea,* it often causes patches of redness or flushing on the nose, cheeks, forehead, and chin. For some people, including Fred, the symptoms of rosacea appear as bumps, lesions, or pimples, and this type is known as *papulopustular rosacea,* which looks similar to acne. Patches of these bumps, which can be pus-filled and which can make some people feel burning or stinging sensations, generally surface in the center of the face. While this type of rosacea may look like acne, it is caused by different factors, and, therefore, may not respond to routine acne treatments.

There is also a form of rosacea that causes a thickening of the skin on the nose. It can manifest as "irregular surface nodules," or it can appear as enlargement of the nose, referred to as *phymatous rosacea.*[7] Additionally, there is a type of rosacea that affects the eyes, known as ocular rosacea, making them red, vascular, swollen, and watery.[8] On occasion, rosacea can emerge as a recurring rash that can be hard to visually classify. In this case, a biopsy of the skin is helpful in determining if the symptoms are, indeed, due to rosacea.

The root causes of rosacea are not entirely known. This condition is thought to be hereditary, although studies have found several other causal factors. Some studies have "suggested that a bacterium commonly associated with peptic ulcers and other gastric disorders, called *Helicobacter pylori,* may cause rosacea in some patients."[9] A weakened immune system is also believed to make a person susceptible to rosacea. A recent study found that a type of mite can proliferate in the skin of people with rosacea when their immune system is impaired, resulting in irritation and outbreaks of rosacea.[10] For this reason, boosting the immune system of those with rosacea through diet and supplement regimens can help improve their condition. Also certain things—notably, stress and sun exposure, as well as spicy foods and alcohol consumption—are known to kick up a bout of rosacea in those who have a propensity for it.

Stress-related rosacea patients often do not see results when they use conventional treatments alone. In Fred's case, we tried topical creams, and they provided only minimal improvement of his condition. As we examined what was going on in his life at the time, we kept coming back to his daughter's nuptials and the related pressure he felt to provide her with a perfect day. He was conscious of the burden he felt, but did not realize the important link between his stress and his rosacea. Fred's experience with stress-related rosacea is quite common. In fact, a large survey conducted by the National Rosacea Society shows that stress is a triggering factor in 79 percent of rosacea cases.[11]

Treatment Options in Rosacea Conditions, Such as Fred's

It is important to reduce your stress in order to curb the negative effects it has on your skin.

If you are experiencing outbreaks of rosacea during or after an emotionally taxing time, it is imperative that you reduce the stress hormones in your body in order to curb their negative effects on your skin. This can be achieved through relaxation exercises that restore balance to your hormonal processes. It could be as simple as incorporating a few minutes of meditation into your daily routine, or indulging in a floating-tank session or a massage on a weekly basis. For more details on the healing powers of meditation and massage, turn to Chapters 5 and 6. Other holistic techniques that are beneficial include acupuncture, psychotherapy, and biofeedback. You can find out more about these therapeutic techniques in Chapters 8, 10, and 12, respectively.

Following a specific diet can help to avert rosacea breakouts, as we know that certain foods can aggravate and activate rosacea. I recommend that my patients avoid alcohol, spicy or hot-temperature food and drinks (like tea or coffee), and also liver, yogurt, sour cream, cheese, chocolate, vanilla, soy sauce, yeast extract, vinegar, eggplant, avocados, spinach, peas or lima beans, and citrus fruits. A good food to add to your diet includes reishi mushrooms which, preliminary research has shown, boost the immune system.

Supplements can help bolster the immune system and fight the bacteria associated with rosacea. Indole-3-carbinol acts as an antioxidant and detoxifying enzyme, which also has anticancer effects. Milk thistle is a beneficial supplement because of the silymarin, a flavonoid complex extracted from the seeds of the thistle that acts as an antioxidant and liver detoxifier. This extract also inhibits inflammatory compounds, which reduces eruptions of rosacea. Other helpful supplements include the prebiotics fructo-oligosaccharides (FOS) and inulin. They are not digested or absorbed in the stomach or small intestine, but are instead only absorbed in the colon where they are digested by bacteria—this can be very beneficial in cases where the bacteria *Helicobacter pylori* plays a part in triggering outbreaks of rosacea.[12] Oil of oregano, a natural antibiotic, is also a suggested supplement. Some dermatologists like to recommend its use as a topical ointment, but I think it is also a good idea to take this as an oral supplement because oregano works to break down bad bacteria in the intestines and on the skin. For more details on diet and supplements that can serve to bolster your immune system, which plays an important part in the outbreaks of rosacea, please refer to Chapter 9.

Light-emitting diode (LED) therapy can also clear the skin irritation caused by rosacea. This therapy penetrates deep layers of the skin and triggers the cells to regenerate, thus breaking down damaged cells and causing new, healthy ones to grow. LED therapy also heals the inflammation, lesions, and wounds associated with rosacea. Light-emitting diode therapy is discussed in more detail in Chapter 11.

For those with rosacea, lasers treatments are beneficial as they can destroy the prominent blood vessels often seen with rosacea. After two to four sessions, the redness can be significantly decreased, relieving people with rosacea of the chronic flushing. The results of laser treatments can last up to one year or longer, although, if the person's rosacea is exacerbated, new blood vessels can appear.

Other helpful treatment options include topical creams, specifically metronidazole, which decreases the bacteria associated with rosacea. Azelaic acid is another topical medication used to treat rosacea, as it functions to kill bacteria and decrease keratin production. There is also a new topical cream, approved by the FDA in September 2013, called brimonidine, which decreases inflammation and shrinks blood vessels. For more information on how topical creams can heal stress-induced skin conditions, please refer to Chapter 13.

Fixing Rosacea Problems

Taking advantage of the treatments discussed in this chapter will help to eradicate the redness and lesions associated with rosacea, and prevent further outbreaks. This was the case for Nita, a sixty-one-year-old Caucasian female with a history of a chronic rash on her face. She visited multiple doctors and was told her rash was due to a myriad of conditions, ranging from lupus to eczema to acne. Surprisingly, her rash had not been biopsied by any of these doctors.

When she came to me, the first thing we did was perform a biopsy of the affected skin where we discovered that she had *papulopustular rosacea* that resembles acne. We discussed changing her lifestyle through incorporating stress-reduction exercises, such as meditation, massage, floating-tank therapy, yoga, and acupuncture, and through boosting her immune system with the nutritional supplements and dietary changes outlined earlier. She also began to use the topical cream metronidazole, which decreases the bacteria associated with rosacea, and took advantage of our light-emitting diode treatments.

She returned to my office a few months later, following her son's wedding. With tears in her eyes, she showed me a picture from the nuptials distinctly showing that her skin had cleared completely. She looked beautiful.

Eczema

Shelly's Struggle

Like most women who juggle a career and kids, Shelly, a fifty-seven-year-old Caucasian woman, could barely find a minute to herself. A typical day in her house began by herding her teens out the door, grabbing breakfast as she ran to her car, and eating on the commute to work. She never had time to go to the gym or properly take care of herself. In fact, most of Shelly's meals seemed to take place in transit, on the drive to meet her clients or pick up one of her kids.

Shelly began motherhood at the age of forty, a little later in the game than some. Now, at fifty-seven, she had clawed her way up the corporate ladder in an advertising firm, dealing with demanding clients at all hours of day and night. Her husband frequently traveled for work, so most nights Shelly felt like a single parent when she got home late from the office to tend to the needs of her teenagers. Shelly's hectic schedule eventually contributed to a scaly, itchy, eruption of eczema all over her face, neck, and chest that made meeting with clients an ordeal. She took to wearing high-necked, long-sleeved dresses and blouses. The steroid creams prescribed by her previous doctor had stopped working on her breakouts.

With inflamed patches of eczema all over her body, and desperate to find a treatment that would work, Shelly came to see me. I told her that topical skin treatments alone are not always sufficient to address stress-related eczema and said she also needed to deal with the chronic stress in her life and learn to manage it. Together, we worked out a treatment plan that addressed both Shelly's eczema and her stress. Amazingly, within three weeks, her eczema began to improve. At her daughter's high-school graduation months later, in the heat of the summer, Shelly wore a sleeveless dress. It was the first time she'd been able to show that much skin in ten years. She felt beautiful.

Medical Analysis of Eczema Conditions, Such as Shelly's

> Stress can trigger the condition of eczema (atopic dermatitis) for those with a predisposition to it.

Eczema comes from the Greek word to boil over. All acute lesions under the general term of eczema typically have the same clinical appearance, that of red, scaly patches of skin, sometimes with tiny vesicles (blisters). Most cases have severe scaling, with swelling and erythema (redness), but if tiny blisters occur, they often rupture and weeping occurs, followed by the formation of a thin crust on the inflamed area after the blisters dry.

The condition of eczema, also referred to as *eczematous dermatitis,* encompasses the larger category of skin disorders, including allergic contact dermatitis. Allergic contact dermatitis is caused when the skin comes into contact with a substance you are allergic to, for example poison ivy. Eczema also refers to irritant contact dermatitis, which is caused when the skin gets aggravated by repeatedly coming into contact with a harsh substance, for example an abrasive soap. The most common type of eczema is atopic dermatitis. This condition is prevalent in about two percent of adults and about ten percent of children. The symptoms include chronic eruptions of itchy, swollen, and flaky patches of skin. The itchiness and discomfort can disrupt sleep, as well as significantly impair the quality of life for those who have this condition. When eczema erupts on the face and neck, as well as other visible areas, it causes social discomfort and embarrassment, and the stress from this scenario often exacerbates breakouts.

What Causes Eczema?

The cause of eczema (atopic dermatitis) is thought to be due, in part, to a genetic mutation in the outer layer of our skin that acts as a barrier to the outside world. This outer layer of skin functions as a permeable boundary to keep good elements inside and harmful elements, such as bacteria, toxins, and allergens, out. When there is a mutation in the filaggrin gene (the filament-aggregating protein), which helps to create the barrier function of the skin, then the skin's ability to act as a protective boundary is compromised.[13] Then, if the skin cannot properly keep harmful elements out, irritants that include harsh cleansers and detergents, industrial chemicals, tobacco smoke, staphylococcal bacteria, and even extreme temperatures, have an easier time entering, and they can trigger bouts of eczema. It is also thought that the weakened skin barrier allows more allergens to enter through the skin, which is why there is a close tie between allergies, such as hay fever and asthma, and eczema. Bacteria is also thought to trigger flare-ups. A recent study conducted at Drexel University College of Medicine in Philadelphia found that "staphylococci bacteria on the skin's surface can produce a biofilm that occludes the sweat ducts, which results in atopic dermatitis and eczema."[14]

Stress and Eczema

For those with a predisposition to it, stress can trigger the condition of eczema (atopic dermatitis). When dealing with stress on a chronic basis, or when life just becomes more stressful due to work, school, home life, family situations, etc., the body reacts by releasing hormones, such as cortisol and adrenocorticotropic (also known as ACTH or corticotrophin), that help it cope with the stress. A study has shown that those with eczema release a significantly higher amount of these stress-related hormones.[15] These increased hormones initiate your cells' inflammatory response, and outbreaks of painful patches of eczema can occur. Because inflamed areas of skin are incredibly itchy, scratching the skin can allow a secondary infection to ensue, and prolong the duration of the outbreak. It is also important to note that flare-ups of eczema can be emotionally and psychologically distressing, which, in turn, worsens the outbreak. A key factor to treating this condition includes preventing the exacerbation of symptoms.

Treatment Options for Eczema Conditions, Such as Shelly's

> Your stress can work against skin treatments until you address it.

If your problem is stress-related eczema, there are multiple treatment options to help your condition. It is important to mention here that prescription medication and cutting-edge technological therapies should always be coupled with holistic methods that address the stress in your life, otherwise the stress will work against the other treatments, and continue to trigger the eczema flare-ups.

In terms of prescription medication, there are several types of topical prescriptions—in cream, spray, foam, or ointment form—that are beneficial in treating eczema. Since this condition is associated with a dysfunction in the skin's ability to act as a protective layer, barrier-repair creams can help reinforce the skin's ability to function as a boundary and keep harmful environmental agents out. Barrier-repair creams can repair and restore the barrier of the skin by supplying water and lipids, a crucial component in the tissue that makes up the outer layer of the skin. Studies have shown that this type of treatment can help to restore the skin's epidermal (outer) function.[16] Other beneficial prescription topicals include anti-inflammatories and calcineurin inhibitors. These products suppress the response of the skin's immune system that is responsible for triggering the inflammatory reaction associated with eczema. For more details on prescription topicals and their benefits, turn to Chapter 13.

Light-emitting diode therapy, which sends a special type of light deep into the skin, serves to reduce the redness associated with eczema that is caused by inflammation and increased blood flow to the lower layers of the skin. To read more about light-emitting diode therapy, turn to Chapter 11.

When treating stress-induced eczema, it is important to incorporate holistic methods that can boost the functioning of your skin's immune system as well as mitigate your stress levels. Adjusting your nutritional intake with the diets recommended in Chapter 9, may also make your outbreaks shorter and assist in a quicker recovery. There are also many beneficial nutritional supplements that will help. Studies have shown the probiotic (*Lactobacillus rhamnosus* GG) intestinal bacteria appear to prevent atopic dermatitis by affecting the person's nutritional status and immune system. They have also shown that the prebiotics and black currant seed oil containing essential fatty acids, specifically all three forms of linolenic acid, can serve to reduce the development of eczema or atopic dermatitis.[17] Linolenic acid (omega-6 fatty acid) reduces the severity of eczema. Zinc is essential for immune function, wound healing, and skin health. Vitamin E moisturizes skin, which can help the impaired barrier layer of the skin that is associated with eczema. Vitamin C prevents the secretion of the compound histamine by white blood cells that triggers the inflammatory response in your skin cells. Vitamin C also increases the breakdown of the compound histamine, which is useful in fighting the inflammation associated with eczema. Another beneficial supplement is quercetin bioflavonoid, a naturally occurring substance that gives many fruits and vegetables their vibrant color, and is effective because of its anti-inflammatory and anti-allergenic properties. This supplement is shown to inhibit the manufacture and release of histamine and inflammatory mediators, which can increase the irritated skin associated with eczema. Fish oils (omega-3's) can reduce allergy and inflammation signs and symptoms as well. And lastly, there is *glycyrrhetinic acid,* a licorice extract that has an effect similar to a topical hydrocortisone treatment and can reduce the redness, itching, and swelling associated with eczema. For more details and specifics on beneficial supplements, turn to Chapter 9.

Incorporating a few minutes of daily meditation along with a weekly or bimonthly massage into your schedule, can reduce the amount of stress hormones in your body, and help alleviate flare-ups of eczema. Breath and movement exercises, such as yoga or Pilates, are also advantageous in alleviating stress. For more details on how mediation, floating-tank therapy, and massage can be used to reduce stress, turn to Chapters 5 and 6. For details on the benefits of acupuncture and biofeedback, turn to Chapters 8 and 12. For information on the benefits of yoga, or for directions on how to incorporate exercise into your life, refer to Chapter 7.

When dealing with stressful life situations, psychotherapy is a useful treatment that can alleviate stress and clear up a consequent stress-related skin condition. For a discussion of the benefits of therapy and the techniques or approaches available, turn to Chapter 10.

RECLAIMING LIFE

The treatments outlined in this chapter can help anyone with stress-induced eczema reclaim their life from the incessant and painful presence of chronic eczema. This was the case for my patient Alexia, a thirty-nine-year-old Hispanic woman, and mother of two. I treated her for eczema and helped get her outbreaks under control. She was doing so well I didn't have to treat any outbreaks for several years. But when marital problems, which included remaining in the same house with her soon-to-be ex for the sake of the children and to conserve financial resources, became hard to handle, the stress of it all eventually landed her back in my office with scorching patches of eczema all over her face and neck. After connecting Alexia with protective services, I recommended that she incorporate stress-management practices into her routine. She began meditation, Pilates, and a massage once a week. I also started her on weekly sessions of light-emitting diode therapy and recommended that she take supplements and use a barrier-repair cream. Within two weeks, she was again feeling better and saw a marked difference in her eczema–the scaly patches were clearing. After seven weeks, her eczema had almost completely gone away and her complicated life was taking a turn for the better.

While not all cases of atopic dermatitis will be cleared with the aforementioned protocol, most cases certainly will be helped. It should be noted that, in some severe cases, more extensive measures, including oral therapies, may be required in order for your atopic dermatitis to go into remission, especially if a bacterial infection, such as *staphylococcus aureus,* has occurred on the eczema-affected areas of the skin. In these cases, you should consult a dermatologist because additional therapy, such as antibacterial washes, bleach baths, and the administration of topical mupirocin through the nostrils, is required.

Shingles—Herpes Zoster

Shana's Burden

It was during a grueling, two-hour commute home in bumper-to-bumper traffic, that Shana, a Caucasian in her early thirties, began to experience a splitting headache. At first, she attributed it to the blinding sun glaring in her eyes, but then the next morning, she awoke with a fever, her head still ached, and there was a strange stinging sensation on her forehead where a rash was developing. Her mom suggested it could be shingles, which Shana dismissed. She'd never even had chickenpox, only the chickenpox vaccine, and you can't get shingles from that, right? Or so she thought... until she did some research. That's when it became clear she had a serious case of shingles that had already spread like wildfire across her forehead and left eyelid, and there was a chance the virus could spread further, into her optic nerve, damaging her eyesight. She immediately sought medical attention.

The first thing Dr. Ablon asked Shana was if she had been stressed out lately, and Shana had to admit she'd been exhausted, overwhelmed, and physically dragging for a week before the symptoms of what turned out to be shingles began to surface. She said it felt as though her body was carrying an invisible boulder and she was buckling beneath it. Until her body gave out, Shana wasn't able to put her finger on exactly what was wrong.

While Shana was reduced to bed rest, her friend and housemate wrote her a hot rent check *for the third time.* This is when Shana began to see the crux of the weight she'd been shouldering. "I peeked into her bedroom and it looked like an episode of *Hoarders,*" Shana recalled. There was a thick layer of trash and clothes were matted and jumbled together on the floor–boots would be needed to tromp through all the filth. Dirty dishes with molding food were sprawled across the desk and dresser surfaces. Empty gallon-size vodka bottles clustered under the desk, and empty wine bottles were strewn throughout the mess.

Now, all the lies, all the bounced checks, all the deceit, and all the excuses finally made sense. It was crystal clear their home life had become unlivable. Her friend had been hiding an insidious addiction, and as she deteriorated, Shana's body had absorbed the toxicity of the situation until it finally came to a breaking point and Shana's body broke down–literally. Sometimes the body knows, even before you consciously know.

As Shana set firm boundaries for her own health and sanity, and insisted that her friend move out, she began to mend. The antivirals Dr. Ablon prescribed helped the blisters go into remission, and thankfully they did not travel into her optic nerve. After a few weeks of rest, her energy had returned and she was back to feeling like her old self.

Note: This story was submitted by Susanna DeSimone

Dr. Ablon's Medical Analysis for Stress-Induced Shingles Cases, Such as Shana's

It is well known that shingles, technically known as herpes zoster, is activated by stress. This is not to be confused with herpes simplex, the herpes virus that causes cold sores, which can also be stress-activated. Shingles, a painful, blistering viral eruption, can only flare up after a person has contracted the chickenpox virus. This is because, even after you have healed from chickenpox, the virus lays dormant in your spinal cord. In times of stress, family issues, illness, compromised immunity, and suchlike, the virus is released and appears as grouped blisters distributed along certain spinal nerve pathways. Shingles can occur at any age, especially in times of duress, but if you are older than sixty, you have a higher risk of developing shingles as well as postherpetic neuralgia, the severe post-outbreak pain that can be associated with the viral eruption.

The onset of shingles feels like burning, itching, or tingling in the nerve pathways, followed by the appearance of blisters that are very painful. In Shana's case, there was a burning sensation, a twinge in her eyebrow, and she had no idea what the pain was indicative of until the blisters appeared a week later.

As the blisters progress, they ooze and weep. In this phase, they are contagious and can pass the chickenpox virus on to those who have yet to be exposed to the virus, or have not had the vaccine. You cannot catch shingles from someone else, only chickenpox. Once you have contracted this herpes-zoster virus, it lies dormant until later when, in times of stress, it rears its head as shingles. After the blisters fill with fluid and ooze, they crust over, and you are no longer contagious. The healing process can sometimes take two-to-three weeks, during which time you will feel exhausted and depleted, and your immune functioning will be lowered.

The blisters associated with shingles tend to manifest in a particular pattern on one-half of the body, in areas where sensory fibers from a spinal nerve, known as the dermatome, meet. When shingles erupt on the chest, the painful rash wraps around your midline in front and in back. When they erupt on your face, the red blisters appear on the midline of your face, forehead, eye, cheek, or jawline, but typically stop at the center of the face. If the blisters appear above your eye, and *especially* on your nose, you must seek treatment immediately as there is a chance the virus could travel into your optical nerve and cause damage to your eyesight.

The pain accompanying an outbreak of shingles can be unbearable. This is particularly true for those older than sixty, since the risk for developing long-lasting discomfort, even after the blisters resolve, goes up dramatically, due to a complication from shingles known as postherpetic neuralgia. Those who develop this often experience severe pain in the affected area, which can be extremely sore to the touch and can interfere with daily activities. The pain lasts longer than the customary few weeks it takes shingles to resolve and can be life-altering. For this reason, it is imperative to treat an outbreak of shingles as soon as the blisters appear. And, after evaluating the risks and benefits, anyone age sixty or older should consider getting the shingles vaccine. In older individuals especially, shingles can have serious and long-term consequences.[18] High-risk younger individuals can get the vaccine as well.

Treatment Options for Stress-Induced Shingles Eruptions

First thing I tell individuals is that the sooner treatment for herpes zoster (shingles) is started, the better. The best way to prevent an outbreak of shingles is before it develops, by modifying your lifestyle in order to reduce your stress.

A combination of medications, cutting-edge treatments, and holistic remedies can be used to shorten the lifespan of the virus and prevent a recurrence.

If you are dealing with shingles, you should begin to take oral antiviral medication immediately, as this will help to abate the pain and discomfort from the infection and reduce the time it takes the blisters to heal. Lidocaine patches can also be used to manage pain, as can oral pain medication, such as ibuprofen.

Cutting-edge treatments for shingles are also useful for treating the discomfort, the lesions, and any scarring that occurs. In my clinical experience, pulsed electromagnetic field therapy (PEMF) can reduce pain, burning, and soreness from the blisters during outbreaks. Light-emitting diode therapy (LED), which uses infrared lasers, has been shown to reduce the pain of the blisters and the possibility of relapse.[19]

I have found clinically that infrared and red LED treatments minimize the duration of the lesions, and ease the pain/tingling/burning that can all be part of the outbreak. To read more about how these treatments aid in healing stress-induced skin conditions, turn to Chapters 11 and 12.

In many cases, the blisters associated with shingles can resolve without scarring, but there are cases, as with the original viral infection of chickenpox, where scars can occur after scratching. Discoloration can also occur where the blisters erupt. For Shana, the aftermath of her shingles infection was distressing. The inflammation from the blisters caused a huge purple splotch of hyperpigmentation (discoloration) on her forehead, and she had a deep scar above her eyebrow where she had picked at a blister. In such cases, non-invasive laser treatments can be used to remove the scar. Also topical lighteners can be rubbed on the skin to clear up any post-inflammatory discoloration. In Shana's situation, within a few weeks of utilizing these treatments, she began to see a marked improvement. For details on products and procedures that can help with scarring, turn to Chapters 13 and 14.

While shingles typically runs its course and then resolves, there is a chance that an individual can develop the complication of postherpetic neuralgia (PHN) that can cause life-altering pain. If PHN does develop, topical anesthetics can help with the discomfort. These include anticonvulsant medications, such as gabapentin, that are used to treat seizures, and antidepressants, such as amitriptyline. The Qutenza patch, which contains capsaicin, a compound from chili peppers, has been shown to improve the pain associated with shingles and PHN.[20]

Currently, the Ablon Skin Institute and Research Center is studying the use of red and infrared LED treatments to both prevent the development of PHN and reduce the pain associated with this condition once it arises. There are also new medications, such as EMA401, on the horizon for the treatment of postherpetic neuralgia.[21]

Holistic measures can be taken to minimize the lifespan of the virus. Studies have found that certain supplements decrease the extent of the herpes-zoster viral infection. These include coenzyme Q_{10}, vitamin E, selenium, and methionine.[22]

Supplements also help fight the exhaustion and lowered immune function associated with the virus. For this reason, I suggest taking calcium, vitamins C and B_{12}, and zinc. To learn more about the therapeutic effects of supplements, turn to Chapter 9.

For years, studies have documented the association between stress and many viral eruptions, including herpes zoster (shingles). For this reason, a vital part of treating shingles is to incorporate relaxation techniques into your daily life to manage your stress. This will help your body heal and regain energy. Managing your stress will serve to ensure that you do not experience a recurring outbreak of this virus (although that is rare), or any other stress-related condition.

For those with stress-induced shingles, the first major change I recommend is incorporating a holistic treatment, such as getting a massage, indulging in a floating-tank session, or practicing yoga on a weekly basis. For more details on how to implement meditation, relaxation, and movement techniques to treat your skin condition, please refer to Chapters 5 and 7. For details on the different types of massage therapy and how massage functions as a stress reducer, please refer to Chapter 6.

When dealing with stressful life situations, psychotherapy is a useful treatment that can alleviate stress and clear up consequent stress-related skin conditions. For a discussion of the benefits of this therapy and the techniques or approaches available, turn to Chapter 10.

Biofeedback therapy also helps to combat stress. It teaches stress-reducing techniques by giving you feedback about the muscle tension, brain waves, and other bodily symptoms that occur when your body is stressed out. With a biofeedback session, you learn how to manage your responses to stress. To learn more about the benefits of biofeedback therapy, turn to Chapter 12.

For anyone who is experiencing the symptoms of stress-related shingles, it is important to see your dermatologist immediately and start prescription medications. Also consider employing the above therapies to manage the stress in your life, which can, in turn, curb the virus in your body and send the eruption back into its dormant state. Plus, if appropriate, consider the possible need for vaccination.

2

Stress and Aging

Aging: Overview

As you age, your genes age as well.

Your body begins aging sometime between your adolescence and your mid-twenties. Generally the aging process is associated with the external signs of wrinkles, sunspots, and sagging skin. This process of aging, the one you witness in the mirror, is a reflection of the cyclical process of cellular turnover—where cells grow and break down and new cells are generated. When cells are young, they rejuvenate at a faster pace, making youthful skin dewy and taut in nature. As you age, your body generates less and less new skin. Your cells turn over at a slower and slower rate. Old skin cells accumulate, leaving the surface of the skin looking sallow. The texture of the skin thins as the proteins that provide the support structure of the skin, collagen and elastin, begin to degenerate and shrivel up. Lines appear and the skin sags.

While extrinsic factors, such as stress, sunlight, smoking and drinking, cause the skin to age, intrinsic factors, also referred to as chronological or genetically programmed aging, such as family history, background, ethnicity, and the normal passing of time, also cause skin to age. Aging serves a protective purpose as it prevents old, damaged cells from replicating, actually shutting those damaged cells down. Telomeres are a key cellular component involved in the aging process of our genetic material. They have been called the biological clock of cells because they essentially govern the lifespan of each cell and indicate when it is time for a cell to stop dividing or die.[1]

Together, both internal and external factors affect the functioning of your skin cells and lead to a thinning of the top and middle layers of the skin called the epidermis and dermis. Extrinsic and intrinsic elements cause the skin to age by slowing the turn over of the top skin layer, the epidermis. This results in a problem with the skin's ability to act as a barrier, and decreases the skin's natural protective ability. These aging factors also decrease collagen and elastic fibers in the dermis, the middle layer of the skin, which causes the skin to appear thin and wrinkled to the naked eye.

The aging you view in the mirror, extrinsic aging, is mostly due to inflammation, and appears as roughness of the skin, a yellowing in color, and a deepening of lines and wrinkles.[2] Where there is a drastic loss in collagen, inflammation can manifest as sun damage. While you have little control over the intrinsic factors that cause your skin and body to age, you can now control the extrinsic factors, and in so doing, you can shape how quickly and dramatically your skin ages.[3]

The Role of Stress in Aging

Stress causes aging by disrupting the body's internal regulatory systems that control the release of stress hormones. Long-term stress, or distress, leads to the impaired functioning of the hypothalamus/pituitary/adrenal axis that presides over your long-term stress response by releasing stress hormones, such as cortisol and stress neurotransmitters, into your body. The hypothalamus is the part of your brain that controls the functions in your nervous and endocrine systems. It sends signals to the pituitary and adrenal glands, and working together in a complex dance, these three organs control the release of stress hormones. Stress can also reduce the functioning of the sympathetic adrenal medullary axis, the innermost part of the adrenal gland. It monitors the short-term stress reaction—the fight-or-flight response—by releasing the stress neurotransmitters epinephrine or norepinephrine into the body. Even though short-term stress can be seen as having a beneficial, protective affect on your body, long-term, chronic stress does the opposite—it ravages your body instead. The effects on your body can be worse than detrimental—they can be fatal. A recent study conducted at Oregon State University's Center for Healthy Aging by Dr. Carolyn Aldwin followed over a thousand men for several years and found that those who felt "over-the-top stressful" were three times more likely to die over the course of the study than those who "rolled with the punches." This study is pending publication in *Experimental Gerontology*.

When first experiencing stress, high levels of cortisol are released, but over time, when the stress becomes chronic, it can actually deplete the amount of cortisol the adrenal glands have to release. This leads to adrenal exhaustion, which leaves a person feeling lethargic and tired. As a result, long-term stress impedes the natural equilibrium your body so desperately seeks.

When stress hormones flood the body, by-products of excess-stress are left behind. Over a long period of time, this causes inflammation. And it is inflammation (like that caused by sun damage) that triggers the aging of the skin. Aging happens as inflammation breaks down collagen and elastin, the proteins that provide the support structure of your skin and keep it looking firm and plump. As the collagen and elastin are fragmented, the skin becomes thinner, more fragile, and, of course, more wrinkled.

While we do know that stress causes people to age, the exact way that stress initiates aging on the skin is still theorized about. It is currently proposed that stress causes the release of neuroactive substances in the epidermis, the outermost layer of the skin, and this release activates the inflammatory process in the skin, which then initiates aging. These effects are reflected in skin by wrinkles, lines, and/or the texture of the skin.

JEN'S STRESS-RELATED AGING SKIN

Jen, a thirty-two-year-old Asian woman, had a very full schedule. She held down a job in the daytime and at night was in a graduate program with immense demands. After class, she composed research papers until the sun peeked into her window in the morning, then scrambled to work, and at night dragged her tired body to class. She recalled that coffee and a frenzied schedule fueled her existence. As a result, she had jitters for half the morning, and when her energy crashed in the afternoon, she forced down more caffeine to stay awake until her night class. In these classes, she often had to consume more sugar and caffeine to pay attention. And all during this time, she constantly worried about her class ranking; it was a perpetual weight on her mind and the driving force in her life.

One morning, after a particularly punishing all-nighter, she looked in the mirror and barely recognized the woman staring back. It seemed as though she had aged ten years in the three years of her graduate program. Her skin was sallow, and she had wrinkles around her eyes where there had never been any before. The texture of her skin had changed too; it looked thinner and leathery. But since she hadn't been sunbathing or tanning, the only culprit she could think of was stress. At this point, she realized she needed help and made an appointment to see me. I agreed with her self-diagnosis and recommended a selection of treatments for her that included exercise, meditation, light-emitting diode therapy, anti-aging creams, and laser treatments. The good news is, even though the stresses of her graduate program remained, after several months of using the treatments I had suggested, she saw a great improvement in the texture of her skin and a lessening in the appearance of wrinkles.

Dr. Ablon's Medical Analysis of Stress-Related Aging Conditions, Such as Jen's

> Stress has destructive effects on the skin.

Of all the destructive, pro-inflammatory and pro-aging attacks on your skin, nothing compares to the negative effects of stress. Jen's story is all too common. Many patients have come to me concerned with the signs of aging on their skin. Once the root causes are unraveled, it becomes obvious that the chronic stress in their lives is speeding up their biological clock. Stress makes your cells age more rapidly—literally. One study found that mothers dealing with the stress of a chronically ill child had shorter telomeres than mothers with healthy children, indicating that their cells were aging quicker.[4] Along these same lines, another study found that a tiny amount of the stress hormone cortisol in a person's system ages them by half a year.[5] If the presence of a small amount of this stress hormone can have aging effects, imagine the toll a large amount of this hormone can take on your biological clock.

The presence of higher levels of cortisol in your body can also undermine your ability to sleep at night. Many of you can probably recall tossing and turning at night, overwhelmed by a never-ending checklist, or a troubling life situation. A lot of what you are experiencing in those moments is the excess cortisol in your body. What's more upsetting is that sleep deprivation is also linked to premature aging. A recent study commissioned by Estée Lauder, that involved sixty women ages thirty to forty-nine, demonstrated that sleep deprivation can lead to premature aging and can increase signs of aging in the skin, including fine lines, uneven pigmentation, and decreased elasticity.[6] A cycle in stress-related aging emerges: You can get so stressed out that you can't sleep, and your lack of sleep not only leaves you feeling tired and more stressed out, but also ages you.

Treatment Options for Stress-Related Aging Conditions, Such as Jen's

> A combination of holistic techniques and cutting-edge products and procedures can be used to heal stress-related aging.

Stress-reduction techniques and contemporary advances in dermatology can curb the effects of aging and reverse many of the external damages. In fact, incorporating a healthy diet and exercise (yoga, stretching, even meditation) into your life, not only helps to heal the body, but may even slow aging. A study conducted by Dr. Dean Ornish, which followed thirty-five men for over five years as they fought prostate cancer, demonstrated that those who adhered to a low fat, plant –based diet high in whole grains, and who exercised at least thirty minutes a day, six days a week, had less progression of their tumors.[7] What's more, their telomeres only increased ten percent over the five years. This suggests that holistic stress-reducing techniques may even help slow the aging process.

Stressful Travel Troubles

This was certainly true for Sherry, a fifty-three-year-old Caucasian woman who had recently moved away from her family in Los Angeles to the Midwest. It had been a good career move, but she found that the long hours and lack of family support wore on her. She traveled every week for work. The frenzy of constantly being on the road, coupled with the solitary lifestyle, took a toll on her body. When she stopped by my office while passing through California for work, I saw she had aged five years in the past four months. Through tears, she relayed that she felt as though she had aged ten years. Her skin was sallow and her wrinkles had deepened. We talked about her taking care of her health and her emotional well-being by addressing her stress. I informed her that no matter how many dermatologic cosmetic treatments she underwent, without also controlling her stress, her skin would not improve significantly. She then agreed to incorporate stress-management techniques into her life, in addition to cosmetic treatments, with excellent results. Her skin took on a good color, her wrinkles softened, and she went about her work feeling less frenzied and more accepting of her solitary status.

If you are experiencing stress-induced aging, incorporating the holistic techniques of meditation and massage, as well as breath and movement exercises, can serve to significantly reduce the stress hormones circulating in your body. Meditation, for example, leads to a state of relaxation where breathing, heart rate, and metabolism decrease. This reduces the physical and emotional consequences of stress, which in turn, reduces the stress hormones, thereby decreasing the activation of inflammation that triggers skin-cell aging.

For details on how to practice various forms of meditation, turn to Chapter 5. Another beneficial stress-reducing technique is floatation-tank therapy. This involves relaxing in a floatation tank filled with Epsom salts. Sixty minutes in a floatation tank creates an ideal environment for meditating and relaxing that reduces stress by calming the mind and body. A description and details on this type of therapy is also found in Chapter 5 on meditation.

Practicing the relaxation techniques known as breath and movement exercises, such as yoga, also serve as a form of meditation that reduces stress hormones. Some people prefer this type of meditation because it is paired with movement, as opposed to a stationary practice. The positive effects of physical activity are significant. In fact, one study found that physical activity seems to prevent the telomere shortening, or cell aging, caused by stress.[8] For more details on the benefits of exercise and breath and movement techniques, turn to Chapter 7.

Comparative studies have shown that, likewise, massage therapy decreases the levels of such stress hormones as cortisol. Again, by decreasing stress hormones, you are decreasing the production of neuroactive agents that lead to inflammation in the skin. Inflammation degrades the structural proteins in the skin, such as collagen and elastin, and this causes wrinkles and sallowing of the skin. To learn more details about the health benefits that massages provide, turn to Chapter 6.

Your dietary choices also influence how quickly your cells age. For details on diets that can help reduce the inflammation that triggers aging, turn to Chapter 9.

Light-emitting diode therapy, which is explained in further detail in Chapter 11, decreases inflammation in the skin. This occurs because LED therapy directly reduces the fragmentation of collagen and elastin in the dermis, the inner layer of the skin. LED treatments result in delaying the skin's aging process.

Laser treatments, such as photorejuvenation, infrared, radiofrequency, and ultrasound technology, can be used to combat aging of the skin as they effectively destroy damaged cells and replace them with new cells. These treatments cause the structural proteins in the skin, such as collagen and elastin, to tighten and stimulate new collagen formation. By interacting with the skin cells, laser treatments function to reverse the signs of aging on the skin. Chapter 14 has more details on non-invasive procedures.

Anti-aging creams or topical medications, including gels, foams, sprays, etc., that utilize cutting-edge stem-cell technology, enzyme technology, and antioxidants, can stimulate your skin's ability to replace old cells with new ones. The aging process, as pertaining to the skin, relates to the cells' abilities to break down old cells and generate new ones. Aging slows this process. These creams can reverse the signs of aging on the skin by speeding up the cellular process of regeneration. In particular, human adipose-derived stem cells (ASCs) have become of special interest in the science of anti-aging because of their ability to suppress inflammation and their potential to differentiate into a variety of skin cells. Once these cells replace damaged cells, they lead to the growth of young, healthy cells, in effect turning back your skin's clock. Topical enzyme therapy functions to replace enzymes on the skin that boost the skin's ability to form a protective layer and to repair cells. Growth-factor technology, also a beneficial type of skin cream, mimics the qualities of young skin by repairing damaged, aging skin.[9,10] For details on how each type of anti-aging cream or topical medication functions, and which type of product to purchase, please turn to Chapter 13.

The aging process can be delayed, and that's the good news in this stress-ridden society where many are experiencing accelerated aging. In order to delay the aging process, however, decreasing the stress in your life is paramount. Anti-aging creams, laser, and light-emitting diode treatments are helpful in the process, but only if they are utilized in conjunction with stress-management techniques.

Menopause, Stress, and Aging

CARRIE'S RECOGNITION

During our appointment, Carrie, a forty-nine-year-old Caucasian woman, said to me, "I should feel rested, but instead I feel tired all the time." Carrie had reached the point in her life where her kids had grown up and moved out of her house. Ironically, she has fewer stressors in her life, yet, due to the menopause-related changes occurring in her body, Carrie felt more stressed than ever before. She explained that her girlfriend had recently purchased a new camera and asked to take a picture of her to test it out. When Carrie looked at the picture of herself, she didn't recognize the old lady staring back. Studying the picture, Carrie felt like she'd aged overnight. She had dark circles under her eyes, her hair looked brittle, her skin sagged, and the wrinkles on her neck reminded her of her eighty-year-old mother's skin–leathery. While Carrie was raising her kids, she was too busy to go to the gym. She was always chasing after the kids, carpooling, walking the dog, etc. But even though her house was now empty, she still wasn't making time to exercise. I suggested that she incorporate exercise into her life on a regular basis, follow specific nutritional guidelines and several cutting-edge skin therapies. Within six weeks or following my suggestions, Carrie not only felt less stressed, but she had also lost ten pounds and looked ten years younger. Carrie informed me that her same friend asked to take her picture again, and this time she said, "Gladly."

Dr. Ablon's Medical Analysis of Menopause-Related Aging Conditions, Such as Carrie's

During menopause, women often feel like they have aged overnight.

Going through the process of menopause, a word that comes from the Greek root words *pausis* (stop or cease) and *men* (month), referring to the ceasing of a woman's monthly cycle, can be incredibly stressful for the body. The effects of menopause are, in fact, similar to the effects of chronic stress on the body. Not surprisingly, during this time, women experience a drastic aging of the skin, which can manifest as increased wrinkles, sagging, and loss of fullness in the face, changes that can often make women feel they have aged overnight.

During menopause, and the period that leads up to menopause, women experience a trifecta of ovary-related changes: decreasing ovulation, thyroid dysfunction, and adrenal dysregulation (impaired functioning of the adrenal gland). When these three hormonal systems start to implode, it creates a perfect storm in the body and increases the levels of the stress hormone cortisol, known to trigger aging in the skin.[11] For women experiencing menopause, the levels of stress hormones can fluctuate from low during the day, to high at night, which can hinder the ability to sleep.[12] Sleep deprivation can also have aging effects on the skin. Additionally, the body's production of the hormones progesterone and estrogen slows, and the loss of estrogen can wreak havoc on the skin, causing wrinkles. Because of the stress hormones released into the body during menopause, the treatment of aging due to menopause is similar to treating stress-related aging. Both conditions benefit from stress-reducing practices.

Treatment Options for Menopause-Related Aging Conditions, Such as Carrie's

Curbing stress hormones can slow the aging process.

If you are experiencing aging due to menopause, it is important to curb the stress hormones raging in your body as these are exacerbating the aging process. Incorporating massage, meditation, floatation therapy, and breath and movement exercises are all good techniques for relieving stress.

Just as with treating stress-related aging, anti-aging creams are beneficial for combating menopause-related aging, as are the cutting-edge techniques of light-emitting diode therapy and laser treatments. Additionally, as women go through menopause, they can utilize holistic methods, such as diet and supplements, and non-invasive skin procedures, to fight the aging process and reverse years of aging.

Menopausal, or pre-menopausal women often lack many nutrients in their diet. During this time, nutrition is a powerful tool that can be used to help balance fluctuating hormones. Women in the pre-menopause state often have high androgen (hormone) levels that can cause acne, irregular menses, and cysts in the ovaries. During menopause, excess androgens can lead to dangerous conditions, such as strokes, cancer, or heart disease, and even disrupt feelings of well-being. A healthy diet should focus on reducing insulin resistance and excess androgens (hormones). A good way to do this is to consume foods with a low glycemic index (a measure of how some refined carbohydrates can raise blood sugar), as these types of foods help reduce the presence of androgens. Consuming organic protein (organic chicken, turkey, or grass-fed beef) lowers androgens as well. Also ingesting foods high in fiber (complex carbohydrates) increases the excretion of testosterone. Following a gluten-free diet has been found to reduce the symptoms of menopause, as well. For more details on a low-glycemic diet and a gluten-free diet, including meal suggestions, turn to Chapter 9.

There are several supplements that can help with menopause symptoms. Flaxseed acts as an antioxidant and contains phytoestrogens, the plant-derived form of estrogen, the female sex hormone. Magnesium reduces stress and fatigue. Vitamin E improves menopausal symptoms, as do maca and hops. Valerian helps with anxiety, stress, and sleeplessness. For a complete list of supplements and their functions, refer to Chapter 9 as well.

Non-invasive skin procedures, such as botulinum toxin, are used to relax facial muscles, soften lines and creases, and lift sagging muscles. When done properly, this type of treatment will not paralyze muscles or portions of the face. Its purpose is to bring back the youthful look of your skin from five-to-ten years earlier.

Injectable fillers are also beneficial as you age, and especially, as you go through menopause because of the loss of volume in the face that results in a sagging of the skin. Through filling skin tissue, these fillers can replace volume, which creates a more youthful appearance. They can't quite turn your skin's clock back by thirty years, but they can turn it back by five-to-ten years.

Photorejuvenation (a non-invasive procedure) can turn the clock back as well. In fact, a new study out of Stanford showed that women who completed around six photorejuvenation sessions throughout the year looked as young as they had five-to-eleven years earlier when they began the study.[13] For more details on non-invasive procedures, turn to Chapter 14.

3

Stress and Hair

Hair Overview

Stress can increase the shedding of your hair.

The impact of stress can be experienced in many different parts of the body. You not only feel stress emotionally, or sometimes erupt with a painful or disfiguring manifestation of stress via your skin, but your hair can also display the toll of stress, as well. Hair grows in a cycle that has three main phases: the growing phase (anagen), the transitional phase (catagen), and the resting phase (telogen). For hair on the scalp, the growing phase, which generally encompasses eighty percent of your hair, lasts for two to three years. Hair then passes through the transitional (catagen) phase for one to two weeks, and then approximately twenty percent of your hair enters the resting (telogen) phase and lasts for several months. There are a myriad of ways that stress can affect your hair-growth cycle. Not only can it trigger hair follicles to sprout, it can also push hair follicles into the resting phase where they shed. The following chapters will examine stress-induced hair loss, hair growth, and the impact that hormonal changes associated with menopause can have on your hair.

Hair Loss

Renee's Nightmare

Renee, a forty-two-year-old Caucasian woman, and her husband divorced when their three daughters were seven, five, and two-years-old. They had been married for fifteen years, and it was a huge adjustment not to have him in their daily lives. Renee found herself scrambling to compensate for his frequent absence in her children's world by hustling to soccer games and ballet classes, while struggling with the debilitating grief over the loss of their relationship. Never mind that, as a lawyer, she still had duties to fulfill at her firm.

Before this ordeal, Renee was often complimented on her thick, wavy hair, which she kept layered and styled at shoulder length—colleagues and clients had frequently compared her hair to that of Rachel's character from the sitcom, *Friends.* Then, one day in the shower, Renee began to notice clumps of hair in the drain. When she examined her hair in the mirror, there were huge thinning spots, and she wasn't sure what to do, to her it felt like she wasn't just losing her hair, but was losing a part of herself. As a lawyer, she was incredibly self-conscious when she had to meet with clients clad in a hat or a scarf because she did not feel that was appropriate professional attire. Renee was desperate to get her beautiful hair back, but she didn't know where to start. That's when she came to see me. After utilizing my recommended treatments, Renee was delighted to see her hair regrow and again become full and thick.

Dr. Ablon's Medical Analysis of Hair Loss, Such as Renee's

> Stress-induced hair loss is one of the most common forms of hair loss that dermatologists see.

Stress-induced hair loss is known as *telogen effluvium.* This condition is one of the most common forms of hair loss that dermatologists see.

Effluvium means outflow of hair respectively, and telogen refers to the stage in the hair growth cycle where the hair falls out—the resting stage in this case. There is not a lot of research explaining how telogen effluvium occurs, but it is known that stress and the hormones released during stress somehow stop the production of active hair-follicle growth, leading to an increase in hairs in the resting phase, and, as in Renee's case, an increase in hair shedding.[1]

The type of hair loss known as telogen effluvium can be triggered in several different ways. When there is a shock to the system, growing hairs are jolted into the resting state, where they shed. Commonly, this shock to the body manifests as severe physical or emotional stress. It can be from such occurrences as: injuries, illnesses, accidents, or surgeries. A sudden change in hormone levels after giving birth can also shock the hair follicles and cause them to shut down, or rest, and then shed. This condition is known as postpartum alopecia. When there is a sudden shock to the system, the hair loss is quick and substantial; usually there is a marked difference one-to-two months after the initial onslaught against the body.

The good news is that this condition is reversible. My mother experienced this type of startling hair loss when she was stricken by a sudden string of illnesses, including meningitis and subsequent peritonitis, septic shock, perforated bowel, and emergency surgery. Over this nine-month period, while she was in and out of hospitals and on respirators, she lost almost all her hair and nearly died twice. During her recovery, I started her on low-level light laser treatments for hair growth and, within three weeks, she again had a full head of hair. She was so happy.

You don't need to experience a shocking catastrophe to have stress-induced hair loss. In fact, persistent, or recurrent, stress can also lead to this condition by gradually causing hairs to transfer from the growing phase into the resting phase, where hairs are triggered to shed. This is because, as studies have shown, chronic stress affects the hair-growth cycle in a negative way.[2] Research with animal models indicates a link between stress and a change in hair follicle biochemistry. This change has an intense inhibitory effect on hair growth.[3] In these types of hair loss cases, there is a slow thinning of the hair across the scalp. Poor nutrition or dieting can also lead to this form of hair loss. Mineral, vitamin, and essential amino-acid deficiencies are also contributing factors to this condition, which is why nutrition and supplements are vital to any treatment of hair loss.

Other types of effluvium (hair loss) happen during a different phase of the hair-growth cycle. Medications, such as chemotherapy drugs, can specifically block hair growth during the growing, or anagen, phase, and can trigger the type of hair loss known as *anagen effluvium* that causes a diffuse thinning of the hair across the scalp. This occurs because chemotherapy drugs inhibit rapid cell growth, which is important as it stops cancerous cells from growing, but chemotherapy also stops noncancerous cells, such as hair follicles, from growing. The onset of this type of hair loss is sudden and fast. Growing hairs are triggered to shed before they enter the resting, or telogen, phase and the stress associated with fighting this type of disease can trigger even more hair loss. Even though hair loss occurs, the follicles are not actually destroyed. Hair will regrow, but permanent changes in the hair texture or color may occur.

In both the aforementioned types of hair loss, there is a diffuse thinning of the hair, especially on the frontal hairline. In some scenarios, the process of hair thinning can be slow and subtle, while in other cases, the process can be swift and drastic where clumps of hair fall out while you are brushing or washing it. Hair loss during the growing phase usually leads to complete baldness, including eyebrows and eyelashes, and the pubic area. In either situation, people often find losing their hair so distressing that the emotional duress itself triggers more hair loss. One study found that hair loss "provokes anxiety and distress more profound" than the severity of the hair loss appears to justify. Their findings reflect how important hair is to a person's identity, and hair's symbolic nature and social significance.[4]

The good news is that all these types of hair-loss conditions are fully reversible. Whether you have experienced a sudden shock to your system, a slow thinning of your hair due to persistent stress, or a quick substantial loss of hair due to chemotherapy, there is hope for restoring health to your hair.

Treatment Options for Hair Loss, Such as Renee's

Hair needs the right vitamins and minerals to grow in a rich, healthy, and vibrant manner.

Because studies have shown that stress can inhibit hair growth, when treating this condition it is important to use therapies that address the constant stress in your life in order to curtail the loss of hair and encourage regrowth. These treatments range from nutritional choices, supplements, and low-level light lasers, to acupuncture, floatation therapy, meditation, and in some cases psychotherapy.

Hair needs the right vitamins and minerals to grow in a rich, healthy, and vibrant manner. Since hair is made up of protein, diets rich in protein are key. Deep-sea fish proteins provide many important nutrients, most specifically omega-3 fatty acids. These essential amino acids are required to maintain healthy hair growth and have been shown to decrease the risk of cardiovascular disease and cancer, and reduce the signs and symptoms of diseases associated with inflammation and allergies. In addition, these essential amino acids have been shown to affect mood and behavior, and improve brain function. I love the supplement Viviscal, which contains a proprietary blend that includes a deep-sea fish protein, and biotin, among other nutrients.

A deficiency of Iron, zinc, vitamins B_6 and B_{12}, and the amino acid L-lysine has been linked to the hair-loss condition of telogen effluvium. Vitamins A, C, E, and folic acid are also important for healthy hair growth. Frequently, many people's diets lack the right amount of these vitamins and nutrients, which is why it is often necessary to begin taking supplements.

In the past, many people got the majority of their iron from red meat, but for those who avoid eating red meat, or any meat, iron deficiency and hair loss can be a real problem. I became iron deficient when I stopped eating red meat and saw the toll it took on my hair. As a result, I add iron supplements to my diet. I do believe that red meat in moderation is fine, and now I eat red meat once a week, although it is grass-fed, with no hormones. It is important to note that taking excessive doses of supplements can lead to toxicity, so it is recommended to consult a nutritionally aware doctor or registered dietician before beginning a new regimen. For more information on dietary choices and nutritional supplements that are beneficial in treating hair loss, please turn to Chapter 9.

To manage stress, acupuncture is an effective treatment option, as it increases blood flow and relaxes the heart rate, which serves to clear stress hormones from the body and restore equilibrium to it. For more details on how acupuncture functions, please refer to Chapter 8.

When dealing with stressful life situations, psychotherapy is a useful treatment that can serve to alleviate stress and clear up consequent stress-related skin conditions. For a discussion of the benefits of therapy and the techniques or approaches available, turn to Chapter 10.

Other stress-management options include incorporating meditation and massage into your schedule. Both of these lead to relaxation, which decreases the physical and emotional strains of stress, and thereby, reduces the amount of stress hormones in your body, which, in turn, decreases inflammation and allows hair follicles to grow. For specific information on the types of meditation you can practice, or for details on the various types of massage therapy and their benefits, please refer to Chapters 5 and 6.

Another beneficial treatment for stress-induced hair loss is low-level light laser treatments. These lasers function to decrease inflammation of hair follicles, which allows hairs to grow. For more details on how these laser treatments work, turn to Chapter 14.

For those who experience loss of hair due to chemotherapy, improvement in hair growth can happen quickly. One of my patients, Noreen, a forty-year-old Hispanic mother of four children, who was battling breast cancer, underwent the type of hair loss associated with chemotherapy. Once her mastectomy and subsequent chemotherapy were completed, I started her on low-level light laser treatments, and supplements. She had been using massage and meditation to manage her stress, but she began to incorporate these stress-busting techniques into her schedule more diligently. She also added acupuncture into her routine. Additionally, she began using a topical spray, Tricomin, a copper derivative that reduces inflammation at the hair root, allowing hair to grow. She had new hair growth within three months.

Hair Growth

Monica's Agony

Monica, a thirty-three-year-old Arab woman, married her husband young and they spent the majority of their twenties determined not to get pregnant before they were ready. Monica was meticulous about taking her birth control pills on time and properly using other precautions. Now, in her early thirties, Monica had the opposite problem—she desperately *wanted* to have a child. At first, she was not worried when it didn't happen right away, as everyone told her the process could take time. Six months after she and her husband began trying to get pregnant, a gnawing feeling started in the pit of her stomach. She wondered, *could something be wrong?* This feeling worsened every month as, like clockwork, her period continued to come. A year later, she still was not pregnant, and the monthly cycle of agony had become unbearable. Over the course of those crucial days on the calendar, she would hold her breath waiting to see the verdict: *Would this be the month?* This process became so miserable that Monica and her husband debated whether to try some of the hormonal treatments that could help with conception. Ultimately however, for a variety of reasons, they decided to stick with the natural method.

At the two-year mark, after trying and trying and not succeeding, Monica began to notice hair appearing in places she had never before had hair. Her chin, nipples, and abdomen all exhibited a marked increase in hair growth. She tried waxing and laser removal, only to find the hair returning with fierce persistency. In fact, the hair grew back thicker, and in new areas.

She came to see me, and together we came up with a treatment plan that addressed both her excess hair growth and her stress. After utilizing the recommended treatments, Monica saw a marked decrease in the presence of excess hair, and not long after that, she gave me the good news that she had indeed become pregnant.

Dr. Ablon's Medical Analysis of Hair Growth, Such as Monica's

> Excess hair growth is a medical condition that can be triggered by stress.

Unwanted excess hair growth, *hypertrichosis,* is a condition triggered by stress, which occurs in both men and women in areas of normal hair growth. During times of duress, the adrenal glands are encouraged to release stress hormones, or catecholamines. When this happens, it is common for the adrenal glands to also release androgens, or male hormones, into the bloodstream. These androgens then lead to increased hair growth, as in Monica's case, and are specifically known as hirsutism, or male-pattern hair growth in women. It is important to recognize that the appearance of excess hair growth is not always stress induced—it can also be related to your ethnic background (i.e. the appearance of a mustache or significant, dark nipple hair). This is known as constitutional, or familial, hirsutism. When evaluating your condition, your doctor should use the Ferriman-Gallwey scale, as it takes into account how prevalent excess hair growth is in terms of ethnicity, which makes the hirsutism (excess hair growth) diagnosis more objective.

Interestingly, as we saw with Monica, her excess hair growth was paired with infertility. This is because often an increase in the prevalence of male hormones not only results in excess hair growth but is also seen in polycystic ovarian syndrome, a condition that causes half the hormonal disorders affecting female fertility and makes up about forty percent of the excess hair-growth cases. In about fifty percent of the excess hair growth cases, after a full diagnostic work-up is performed, the triggering factor remains unknown, aside from the continual stress a person is under. In these cases, a combination of treatments can be used to not only fight the unwanted hair growth, but also to alleviate the high stress levels. It is important to note that about ten percent of cases of excess hair growth are due to adrenal tumors and disorders, thyroid tumors, disease, or drug-induced excess hair growth. This could be from oral steroid hormones, glucocorticoids, some antibiotics, oral contraceptives, and certain cardiac medications. For these reasons, full work-ups, or blood tests, should be completed to determine the cause of this condition. Also, I do not recommend removing the excess hair growth until a diagnosis is complete, and the cause of the excess hair growth is determined. Often, treating the causal factor will remedy the excess hair growth, with no need for its removal.

Treatment Options for Excess Hair Growth

> Stress-reducing practices help to decrease the release of hormones that fuel excess hair growth.

Chronic stress can cause an endocrine imbalance and an increase in male hormone, or androgen, production. Engaging in stress-reducing practices will help decrease the release of these hormones. For this reason, incorporating a massage or meditation or pulsed electromagnetic therapy into your regular routine can lessen the amount of stress hormones in your body and return your hormone levels to equilibrium. When you experience continual stress for long periods of time, the liver loses its ability to process these stress hormones, so instead of removing them from the body, they are returned to the blood, which prolongs the excess hair growth. Consequently, supplements that improve liver processing are vital in the treatment of excess hair growth. The nutritional choices you make are also an important factor in treating this condition, and it is important to avoid diets rich in refined carbohydrates, as these foods can fuel excess hair growth.

LORENA'S STRESS-INDUCED HAIR GROWTH

Another of my patients, Lorena, a forty-seven year-old, Hispanic mother of two, experienced stress-induced excess hair growth. At first, she noticed that her abdominal hair had darkened, and this was followed by an increase in the appearance and darkness of her mustache. Initially, she thought it was due to her birth control pills worsening her melasma, or dark pigmentation patches, but as more dark hairs appeared along her jaw line, she began to get worried. Lorena had no menstrual irregularities, or any other symptoms. We drew blood to test for the condition of hirsutism (excess hair growth), and her hormone values appeared relatively normal, although her level of androgens was slightly elevated. We also ordered an ultrasound to look for polycystic ovaries, and were able to rule that out as a causal factor. After this work-up of tests proved that the cause of her hirsutism was idiopathic (of unknown origin), as stress-induced hair growth often is, I probed regarding the stressors in her life. Lorena revealed that her sister had recently been diagnosed with thyroid cancer, and that her father was struggling with dementia. She admitted to feeling more stressed than ever before. So much so, that her appetite had decreased, and she had been unable to sleep.

To combat Lorena's stress-induced hair growth, we came up with a nutrition plan that increased her caloric intake, but kept her on a low-carbohydrate diet. We also added nutritional supplements into her daily diet. Additionally, she and I made out a schedule to increase the amount of exercise she was getting and to add meditation into her regular regimen. It was difficult for her to fit a massage into her schedule, but she was able to do it every two to three weeks.

Within two months, Lorena's excess hair growth had started to decrease. She reported that she felt much better, and was able to deal with the health issues of her family members in a calmer manner. When Lorena followed up with me six months later, she had gained muscle, and looked healthier than ever. She said her life was still hectic, but she was dealing with everything in a more rational and peaceful way.

To utilize the same type of treatments that Lorena did, begin by incorporating stress-reducing activities into your schedule on a regular basis. This could be meditating for five minutes a day, or unwinding with floating-tank therapy, practicing yoga on a regular basis, or getting a massage as often as possible. For details on how to meditate, and information on different forms of meditation, including floating-tank therapy, please turn to Chapter 5. To learn about the healing effects of massage, turn to Chapter 6. For more information on varying types of breath and movement practices, turn to Chapter 7.

Following a low-carbohydrate diet is also an important aspect of combating excess hair growth, as is adding supplements that improve the liver's ability to remove excess toxins and hormones. The amino acids arginine, cysteine, and methionine are beneficial in this regard, as is the supplement milk thistle with silymarin that serves to protect the liver and restore liver cells. Lecithin (a natural byproduct of the liver) is also a helpful supplement; it cleanses the liver and removes fatty liver deposits, as does beta-carotene. The mineral selenium has antioxidant properties, and may also help protect your cells from damage. Beneficial vitamins also include women's formulas that contain phytoestrogens; these serve to counterbalance the increased male hormone production that can trigger excess hair growth. Additionally, vitamins C and E are helpful in fighting this condition.

Another useful supplement is DHA, a type of polyunsaturated fatty acid, which helps to inhibit the process that causes more hair growth. This substance can be found in omega-3 fish oil capsules, or can be gleaned from eating salmon, sardines, or tuna. Evening primrose oil contains a type of polyunsaturated fatty acid that serves the same purpose. Other helpful extracts include serenoa repens, which fights oily skin and hair growth on the body, and royal jelly extract. For more information on how to incorporate a low-carbohydrate diet into your life, as well as for more information on the healing powers of supplements, turn to Chapter 9.

There are beneficial non-invasive procedures and prescription creams that can be used to treat excess hair growth. These include laser hair removal, and the topical cream, Enflornithine, which reduces the speed of hair growth, and can even thin the hair. For more details on how prescription creams and non-invasive procedures work to heal hair conditions, turn to Chapters 13 and 14.

Sonia's Successful Recuperation

The above-mentioned treatments were helpful to my patient Sonia, a forty-one-year-old Caucasian woman, who came to see me for a follow-up appointment after she had undergone a single mastectomy for breast cancer. Remarkably, she had maintained a positive outlook throughout that ordeal, and was in good spirits when she came to see me. Although Sonia was recovering, both physically and emotionally, she was still under a lot of life's pressures. She was incredibly busy taking care of her three children, ranging from ages three to twelve, in addition to her husband, two dogs, a cat, and a bird.

Besides the loss of hair on her head, which was slowly returning, Sonia complained of excess facial hair that was visible when she looked in the mirror. I recommended that she begin mediating on a daily basis and incorporate massage and acupuncture into her routine to decrease the level of stress hormones in her body.

I also suggested she add supplements and follow specific nutritional guidelines to balance her hormone and protein levels. After incorporating these treatments into her life, Sonia's excess hair growth on her face began to dissipate, and she discovered that mediating for five minutes, twice a day, did wonders for her spirit while she continued her recovery process from the cancer treatments. Psychotherapy, in this situation, was also beneficial in dealing with the fear that comes with having to deal with cancer.

Menopause and Hair Loss

Debbie's Distress

Debbie, a fifty-five-year-old Caucasian woman, had long raven hair that had defined her ever since she was a young girl. When she was twelve-years-old, she chopped it off to her chin, then spent the rest of the year depressed until it grew out. As an adult, Debbie felt like her mane had become an extension of her personality. Around the age of fifty, when she began to go through menopause, her hair started to thin out. She didn't want to cut it short, but was eventually forced to chop it off in an attempt to mask her hair loss. At fifty-four, Debbie cringed when she looked in the mirror and saw more scalp than hair. She tried everything to stop this process, from over-the-counter Rogaine to specialty shampoos, but nothing worked. She even went so far as to shop for wigs. To Debbie's dismay, she discovered that most wig hairstyles were short, and designed in such a way that they did not look real or represent her personality. Depression began to set in over the change in her appearance. Ever since her divorce several years before, Debbie's sister had been trying to set her up on a date. Debbie always made excuses as to why she was not available, but the real reason was that she couldn't bear the thought of going on a date sporting a short wig in the style of a bob. At a total loss over what to do, Debbie sought me out. After several months of integrating a number of my suggested holistic treatments into her routine, in addition to cutting-edge treatments, Debbie began to see new hair growth, and has begun to consider going out on one of the dates her sister wants to arrange for her.

Dr. Ablon's Medical Analysis of Menopausal Hair Loss, Such as Debbie's

> At least thirty percent of women complain of hair loss by the age of thirty, and fifty percent of women complain of hair loss by the age of fifty.

Hair loss is a frequent issue women face. At least thirty percent of women complain of hair loss by the age of thirty, and fifty percent of women complain of hair loss by the age of fifty. This dramatic increase demonstrates how hair loss becomes an especially prevalent issue during menopause as women's bodies change significantly. Menopause occurs when the process of ovulation ceases, and hormone production decreases. The hormonal changes during this time trigger hair loss, which can be amplified by chronic stress. For example, hormonal changes, such as a decrease in the body's production of progesterone, lead to hair loss, which is exacerbated by the presence of the stress hormone cortisol, as it can block the progesterone receptors responsible for hair growth. Less progesterone in the body results in an increased production of an adrenal steroid called androstenedione. The presence of this hormone precursor is the main cause of female-pattern baldness. During menopause, chronic stress can also increase the release of the stress hormone cortisol, to the point that the adrenal glands can no longer keep up production, and this leads to a sluggish thyroid, which also triggers hair loss.

Undergoing this menopausal change can be a very stressful experience for women, both physically and emotionally. The media bombards women with unrealistic standards of beauty, particularly the ideal that women should retain their youthful looks—forever. This places a lot of pressure on women as they age, especially since women are staying in the workforce until later in life. Therefore, even as women are going through menopause, they feel compelled to keep up with their younger counterparts in both their looks and all the other aspects of the job. The pressure to live up to society's ideals of beauty often compounds the stress women feel during menopause.[5]

It has been noted that once women have gone through menopause, and the hormones have calmed down or ceased to exist, they feel less stress. [6] However, the stress they still do experience can lead to an increase in stress hormones, which can, in turn, result in a worsening of hair loss. For these reasons, reducing stress during and after menopause is crucial to treating hair loss.

Treatment Overview for Menopausal Hair Loss

> Holistic therapies can treat hair loss due to menopause.

Hair loss due to menopause can be treated with a variety of holistic measures, such as acupuncture, meditation, massage, breath and movement exercises, and diet and supplements. There are also cutting-edge techniques, and medications are available.

COMBATING CANDACE'S HAIR LOSS

Menopausal hair loss was the case for my patient, Candace, a fifty-two-year-old black woman, who loved her work in the movie business, even though she frequently had ten-hour days and survived on as little as six hours of sleep per night. As she underwent the transformation associated with menopause, her menses came about every six months, and she struggled with feeling tired and frustrated. The hair on the top of her head thinned noticeably due to the hormonal changes associated with menopause, and also because of the chronic stress from her work. Candace felt embarrassed about her appearance, and wished her hair looked like that of the young women she worked with, so she began to wear a wig. For five years, Candace donned a wig daily. She wore the wig to work, to the gym, even at home in front of her husband. Frustrated with her appearance, Candace went to multiple physicians who performed many tests to see if she had a thyroid issue or was iron-deficient. When the tests showed that Candace's thyroid and iron levels were within normal limits, she wasn't sure what steps to take next. Candace confessed her dilemma to a friend who suggested that she see me.

I recommended that Candace reduce her stress. She took my advice and incorporated stress-management practices into her routine by taking yoga classes, and buying a book on meditation. She also scheduled a bi-monthly massage. To address possible nutrient deficiencies, I had Candace make adjustments to her diet by incorporating more iron-based nutrients into her meals. She also began to take the hair-strengthening supplement, Viviscal, twice a day. Additionally, she used a biomimetic peptide topical and Tricomin spray, a copper-based spray for the scalp, on a daily basis, and she got corticosteroid injections in her scalp once a month. As part of her treatment, Candace also underwent low-level laser therapy on a weekly basis.

After three months of these therapies, Candace showed significant improvement, and tears welled up in her eyes when she discussed her new hair growth. In fact, Candace reported that she felt better and happier overall. While the female-pattern baldness that Candace experienced is a continual progression of hair loss, with continued therapy, new hair growth can be achieved, and hair loss slowed.

To utilize the same treatments as Candace, you can incorporate the stress-management practices of meditation, massage, acupuncture, and breath and movement exercises into your routine. For details on these practices, turn to Chapters 5, 6, 7, and 8.

The foods you consume affect the health of your hair. For this reason, proper nutrition is an important factor when combating hair loss. In fact, a deficiency in the minerals iron and copper can cause, or exacerbate, the loss of hair. This is why it can be beneficial to consume foods rich in lysine (an essential amino acid responsible for transporting iron), such as meat, poultry, eggs, fish (cod and sardines), and vegetables. Iron can also be gleaned from leafy greens and grass-fed beef. Copper can be found in meats, poultry, eggs, nuts, seeds, and grains. The nutrients you consume can help in metabolizing hormones, which is important during menopause. Brussels sprouts and kale are known to help metabolize estrogen. Following a gluten-free diet also has advantageous effects on your body while you undergo menopause. For specifics on the gluten-free diet, turn to Chapter 9.

Specific supplements are beneficial for the health of your hair. Nutrients such as selenium and zinc promote healthy hair growth, and can be taken in supplement form, as can copper, vitamin D, and omega-3 fatty acids, which your body needs to grow hair. Other helpful supplements include evening primrose oil, which blocks the body from converting testosterone into dihydrotestosterone, a potent hormone that triggers hair loss. Viviscal is a vitamin supplement that can promote hair growth in just three months. To gain more knowledge on the benefits, and uses of supplements, turn to Chapter 9.

Many of my patients have had great results with the cutting edge treatment of low-laser light therapy. This involves using lasers to stimulate the follicles to regrow hair. For more details on how this therapy functions, turn to Chapter 14.

I begin treating hair loss with holistic methods and cutting-edge treatments for the initial six months. These beginning treatments also include the use of Tricomin copper spray, which reduces inflammation and allows hair follicles to grow, and the use of corticosteroid injections directly into the areas of hair loss to stimulate the hair follicles to grow.

After six months, if the hair loss is not resolving or reversing, I then add in medication taken by mouth as a last resort. The first type of oral medication I would have the patient consider is the prescription spironolactone, and following this with the topical medication, minoxidil, which can be obtained over the counter in the form of shampoo. In rare cases, as a last line of action, I would have my patient consider taking the oral medication finasteride. If you are experiencing hair loss that has not responded to any other treatment, then consult a dermatologist to see if your condition calls for these types of medication. New therapies for hair loss are currently under investigation. For more details on these medications and to learn more about possible side effects, turn to Chapter 13.

4

Stress and Nerves

An Overview of Nerves

> Prolonged periods of stress cause many of the stress-related health issues people face today.

In today's society, many people experience prolonged periods of stress, which is why there are so many cases of stress-related health issues. Long periods of stress can wear down your nervous system. The nervous system is made up of the brain, the spinal cord, and an intricate network of neurons. Together, these all function to send, receive, and interpret messages from throughout your body.[1] The autonomic nervous system is that portion of the nervous system regulating messages you don't have control over—the ones that happen automatically—your heart beating, for example. This section of your nervous system reacts when you feel stressed. It has two parts—the sympathetic nervous system and the parasympathetic nervous system. The sympathetic nervous system releases hormones to cope with acute stress, and the parasympathetic nervous system relaxes your system and rebalances your body, but a constant release of stress hormones into your nervous system overrides this parasympathetic nervous system and throws your body off balance, with harmful repercussions.

The body was not designed to handle high amounts of stress for long periods of time. Instead, it was intended to handle the stress of early civilization, such as a roaring lion charging. This type of danger prompts the sympathetic nervous system to release the hormone epinephrine, or adrenaline, triggering the body to respond by either running from the threat, or fighting the ferocious lion head-on, and this active response helps alleviate the stress hormones in the body. In early times, stressors were primarily short-term, and the stress hormones were triggered and released. Today, however, you have emotional stressors, such as losing your job, having a frustrating boss, or attending to the needs of your crying kids on top of long workdays, for prolonged periods of time. If you are constantly under stress, you have a constant release of stress hormones into the body, particularly the hormone cortisol, and exposure to these hormones for any extended amount of time can have deleterious effects on your nervous system.

This can be especially harmful if you are not taking steps to alleviate your stress-hormone levels, either through working out or through other holistic measures, such as getting a massage or practicing meditation. These are therapeutic actions that trigger a response from the parasympathetic nervous system to relax the body and return the nervous system to equilibrium. The following chapters will examine how stress-induced nerve issues can lead a person to experience migraines and/or Bell's palsy.

Migraines

ANGELA'S ACHES

As Angela, a twenty-eight-year-old Asian woman, drove her daughter to kindergarten, a dull, throbbing sensation began to reverberate on the left side of her head, indicating that a doozy of a migraine was imminent. Like a train gaining momentum as it chugs down the track, Angela knew she was on a collision course with a debilitating headache, and hoped she could make it home before feeling its full force. Since Angela's husband, Mark, had been laid off, the migraines had started recurring more and more frequently. They came on swiftly and were overpowering in nature, forcing Angela to lie down in a dark room with a cool cloth on her head and grit her teeth until the throbbing passed. While lying down, she couldn't stop worrying about what they would do in the wake of her husband's layoff. Her paycheck only covered half the mortgage, her husband's unemployment was running out, and they were sinking financially. But even these terrifying what-if scenarios that kept circling through her head were eventually numbed out by the overwhelming thudding sensation on one side of her head. Just as Angela could not come up with a solution for their financial crisis, she also could not escape the onslaught of her migraines. The pills she had been prescribed did nothing to alleviate the severity of these episodes. That's when she came to see me and I gave her several stress-management techniques and cutting-edge therapies to try. After several months, Angela happily reported back to me that she had a better sense of well-being and her migraines were occurring far less often.

Dr. Ablon's Medical Analysis of Stress-Induced Migraines, Such as Angela's

> Stress-induced migraines can severely impact your daily life.

A migraine is an intense headache with a throbbing pain, oftentimes felt near the temples or behind an eye or ear. The pain can be so intense it leads to nausea and vomiting. Sensitivity to light and sound is common, followed by temporarily seeing spots or losing your vision. Migraines can last a few hours or a few days, and tend to occur more frequently during times of stress. While not life-threatening, they can severely impact your daily life and impede your ability to go to work, tend to your family, or take care of pending responsibilities, and can even render you bedridden. There is a high incidence of Americans with debilitating migraines, as noted in Jane Brody's *New York Times* article, "28 million Americans suffer from severe migraines that leave them temporarily unable to function."[2]

Studies have yet to fully explain what causes stress-related tension migraines, although it is believed there is a hereditary disposition for this painful condition. Recent discoveries also indicate that stress-related migraines are due to an underlying disorder of the central nervous system that sets off neurological and biochemical changes that, in turn, increase stress hormones.[3] This increase in hormones causes inflammation, which initiates blood vessels to swell and put pressure on the surrounding nerves, resulting in pain. Recent studies also show how stress can cause the release of peptides, or protein fragments. These peptides can trigger the blood vessels to dilate, which, in turn, stimulate an inflammatory reaction and rile up the nerve cells, causing a chain reaction of pain to travel up and down the nerve pathways in the brain.[4]

Emotional stress is a large factor in triggering migraine episodes, regardless of whether you inherited a gene for this condition or have a disorder of the central nervous system. Other triggering factors can include abnormal levels of neurotransmitters, such as serotonin that promotes sleep and overall emotional well-being, dopamine, or stress hormones. High levels of these elements have been found in people with tension headaches. It is also thought that low levels of magnesium in the body can cause nerves to misfire, and this too can be a factor in the onslaught of stress-related migraines. Further, the presence of too much nitric oxide, a molecule that is an important biological regulator, has also been suggested as a trigger for migraines. And studies have also shown that estrogen fluctuations during adolescence and adulthood can lead to tension migraines.

Treatment Options for Stress-Induced Migraines

To treat stress-induced migraines, begin to incorporate stress-reducing techniques into your life.

If you have stress-related migraines, relief can be found through a comprehensive treatment plan that includes holistic therapies, cutting-edge techniques, and non-invasive procedures.

JAMES'S JARRING STRESS

My patient James, a fifty-three-year-old African-American father of six children, originally came to see me for a routine skin exam and then began to discuss the frequent migraines he was incurring. He and his wife both worked fulltime, and with a packed house of kids at home, the pressures on them were immense. James felt stress from multiple directions, prompted by arguments with his boss, his wife, and his kids. Often, he said, he experienced tension headaches that usually started out as a dull ache in the back of his neck and over his eyebrows, then turned into a pressure, like a thick rubber band squeezing his head, and left him exhausted and depleted. I told him these were migraine episodes, and I discussed with him the importance of managing his stress. This is important, I told him, in order to relieve the tension that can build up in his body, and reduce the stress hormones that subsequently get released and can act as a triggering factor in his stress-induced migraines. I also suggested avoiding certain foods that can initiate migraines, and incorporating supplements to help inhibit some of the chemical processes involved in causing migraines. A few months later, after utilizing the therapies I suggested, he was pleased to report that the frequency and severity of his migraines had lessened dramatically.

If you are experiencing stress-induced migraines, you should immediately begin to incorporate stress-reducing techniques, such as meditation, into your life. This can be as simple as meditating for five minutes in the morning and five minutes at night. As a form of meditation, you can also try floating-tank therapy, which suspends you in a tank of Epsom salts with all other stimuli removed. This allows for a calm, meditative state that reduces the effects of stress hormones. Breath and movement exercises, such as yoga, can also relieve stress, as can incorporating other types of exercise into your life. For more details on different forms of meditation or breath and movement exercises, turn to Chapters 5 and 7.

Getting a massage, especially a scalp massage, can serve to reduce muscle tension and stress, particularly when incorporated into your schedule on a regular basis. Inhaling lavender oil, which can be integrated into a massage, or simply rubbed on the temples, neck, or shoulders, has been found to reduce the severity of migraines.[5] Aromatherapies with such oils as lavender appear to increase relaxation and have a calming affect. In my office, I frequently use this technique to calm individuals before procedural treatments. To read more about aromatherapies and the healing effects of massages, see Chapter 6.

Acupuncture is also a beneficial treatment, as studies have found that it can reduce the pain associated with migraines, and even prevent the occurrence of this debilitating condition. In fact, one study, published in the *British Medical Journal,* followed a group of test subjects who used acupuncture, in addition to standard medical care, to treat their chronic headaches or migraines, and another test group who did not use acupuncture, but only standard medical care to treat their chronic headaches or migraines. Over the course of three months, the group of patients who used acupuncture to treat their migraines experienced significantly fewer headaches throughout the year.[6] To learn more about acupuncture and how it works, turn to Chapter 8.

The foods you consume can also be a triggering factor in the onslaught of a migraine. If you are racked with stress-induced migraines, avoid alcohol, especially red wine. Avoid caffeine as well, along with foods containing nitrates, such as deli meats and hot dogs. Additionally, avoid foods with the naturally occurring substance tyramine, which can be found in aged cheese, soy, hard sausage, smoked fish, and fava beans, and do not consume foods that contain the flavor enhancer monosodium glutamate (MSG), or the artificial sweetener, aspartame.

Supplements you should consider adding to your diet include flaxseed oil and/or fresh crushed flaxseed, both rich in omega-3 fatty acids that can act as an anti-inflammatory. Fresh ginger can also inhibit inflammation and act as an antioxidant, as can the herb feverfew, which contains substances that help to inhibit the dilation of blood vessels. As shown in studies, adding magnesium as a supplement has also been beneficial in reducing the onslaught of migraines, especially since low levels of this mineral can lead to stress, insomnia, and PMS.[7] Riboflavin (B_2) and S-adenosylmethionine can help with chemical processes in the brain. For more details on the many benefits of supplements, turn to Chapter 9. If you are taking prescription medications, it is important to remember that supplements can interact with some of them, so you should check with a nutritionally aware physician before incorporating supplements into your diet.

Cutting-edge therapies are helpful in treating migraines, especially if you're looking for techniques to relieve the pain associated with migraines aside from prescription medication. Pain relief can be had from pulsed electromagnetic-field therapy (PEMF), light-emitting diode (LED) therapy, and biofeedback. These therapies can decrease muscle tension and the pain associated with migraines. To administer treatments at home, you can buy a PEMF device, which delivers short pulses of painless electrical currents to the affected area. To learn more about how PEMF therapy functions, turn to Chapter 12 on electrical stimulation therapies.

Biofeedback teaches stress-reducing techniques by giving you feedback about the muscle tension, brain waves, and other bodily symptoms that accompany migraines while they are occurring. When your body is stressed, blood vessels constrict and blood flow to the main organs becomes limited. With a biofeedback session, you learn how to manage the blood flow to the brain and thereby reduce the pain of stress headaches. This is a great alternative for those with recurring stress migraines, as studies have found it can reduce the frequency and duration of these migraines.[8] To learn more details about biofeedback therapy, turn to Chapter 12.

Ultraviolet LED therapy can also help with migraine-associated pain. Ultraviolet or red LEDs can decrease the inflammation related to migraines and thereby relieve the accompanying pain. Studies in this regard are just beginning, but it is believed that LED therapy works by blocking pain-transmitting chemicals, and by triggering endorphin production to help with pain relief. This therapy also helps to improve lymphatic drainage, reduce swelling, and increase DNA and RNA synthesis to replace damaged cells. To learn more about how LED therapy functions, turn to Chapter 11.

There is also the option of using botulinum toxin injections to treat stress-induced migraines—studies have shown that this treatment helps to reduce the frequency and severity of migraines.[9] Although studies have yet to fully explain why this treatment works, when I use this treatment in my office for my patients with stress-induced migraines, the results are significant.

Palsies

My Own Nightmare (Dr. Ablon)

I awoke to a loud buzzing sound grating in my ears, and numbness in my face—I knew something was off in my body. *Perhaps I have a migraine coming on,* I thought. I gingerly eased out of bed, and padded into the bathroom. When I looked in the mirror, I gasped. The left side of my face drooped oddly. I gently prodded my cheek with my finger, and could not feel any sensation. When I tried to smile, the right side of my mouth curved upward while the left side of my mouth remained in place. Worried that I had suffered a stroke, I tried to scrunch my eyebrows and move my forehead. I couldn't move my forehead, which was good news in a way, for if I could have moved my forehead, that would have indicated that I had, indeed, had a stroke.

Waking to find the left side of my face paralyzed was extremely alarming, and, frankly, quite humbling. Every day, I would do battle with myself in the mirror as I looked at my reflection and tried to move the paralyzed part of my face, to no avail. I finally understood the struggle that my patients with facial paralysis or a severe disfiguring asymmetry confront every day. After spending two weeks at home, avoiding all human contact, aside from my family, I gave in and went back to work. I wore glasses to cover my weird stare, thinking that would make patients feel more comfortable, but really, it was for my own comfort. I used my hand to cover my mouth, and sometimes taped my forehead back to even out my drooping skin. One day, I had a patient actually tell me she didn't want me to do Botox on her if it would give her a look like I had around my eye. I explained to her that I had Bell's palsy, but I'm not sure she really understood. For a doctor working in the world of aesthetic medicine, I had been brought to my knees–ultimately, it was a wakeup call. Stress affects everyone. No matter what your specialty is, your body can only take so much. My body had, in fact, been sending me small signals for some time to let me know that I was under too much stress, but with the onslaught of Bell's palsy, it was *screaming* at me. I knew it was vital that I reduce my stress and change my lifestyle.

Determined to fight this condition, beat it, and, if necessary (as there is no guarantee of a full recovery from Bell's palsy), deal with the residual symptoms, I used everything in my power to recover as quickly as possible. I began by incorporating stress-management techniques I always recommended to my patients, such therapies as meditation and massage, into my regular routine. I cut out foods that trigger inflammation, and I utilized acupuncture and light-emitting diode therapy to reduce inflammation. In three weeks, I had the first sign of movement on my upper right eyelid. Five weeks into my recovery, my face was almost back to normal, except for some residual ear pain and blurred vision, which occurred, along with fatigue, late in the day (something I had never experienced prior to the Bell's palsy). Six weeks into my recovery, my facial paralysis had resolved, and I was filming segments for the daytime talk show, *The Doctors,* although I was still concerned that my face would appear asymmetrical on camera. After viewing the footage, I was relieved to see I looked like my old self.

Ultimately, I owe a lot to my disorder. Becoming disfigured, albeit for a short period of time, helped me become more empathetic toward those with any sort of disfigurement, and my journey to recovery inspired me to write this book. I bring my experiences and techniques for healing to you, the reader, to help you fight the fight toward restoration.

Dr. Ablon's Medical Analysis of Stress-Related Bell's Palsy

> The link between stress and the development of Bell's palsy cannot be overlooked.

Bell's palsy is caused by damage to the facial nerve that controls muscles on one side of the face, and results in paralysis or weakness in the muscles on that side of the face. When the muscles droop on the side of the face that is affected, it leads to loss of muscle function in the forehead, eye, cheek, mouth, and chin muscles. An inability to close the eye leads to dry eyes and irritation requiring immediate attention to prevent permanent damage and visual disturbances.[10] While viral and bacterial infections, tumors, trauma, or medication can all ignite Bell's palsy, the link between stress and the development of this debilitating condition cannot be overlooked. Even though studies have yet to find a direct causal relationship between stress and Bell's palsy, they have shown that "psychological stressors are prevalent in patients with facial paralysis."[11,12,13] And certainly, in my own experience with Bell's palsy, stress was an indisputable instigating factor.

Stress can lead to Bell's palsy by causing inflammation and immune-system depression. This combination allows dormant viruses to be awakened to attack the nervous system. In the case of Bell's palsy, a virus assails the facial nerve, causing inflammation, swelling, and paralysis of the nerve that supplies muscle movement to the face. Symptoms tend to worsen over the first week and then start to resolve at around the third or fourth week. In many cases, symptoms can persist for up to three or four months. In occasional cases, palsy or hearing damage is permanent.

Treatment Options for Stress-Related Bell's Palsy

If you are experiencing stress-induced Bell's palsy, the facial paralysis can be treated through a myriad of therapies that are effective in managing the stress you are under, thereby healing your symptoms.

Holistic therapies can help reduce the harmful hormones associated with stress. These include utilizing meditation on a daily basis, or incorporating floating-tank therapy into your regular routine. Massages can also alleviate stress hormones and serve to reduce inflammation. For more details on these holistic alternatives, turn to Chapters 5 and 6.

Other holistic avenues for healing include incorporating nutrients into your diet that can help your nerves recover from the damage caused by Bell's palsy. This includes adding nutrients that are rich in vitamin A, such proteins as eggs or whole mild liver, or taking the supplement beta-carotene (your body can convert this substance into vitamin A). Also, foods filled with copper, such as nuts, beans, potatoes, dark leafy greens, cocoa, and dried fruits, are beneficial. Vitamin B_{12} is another helpful supplement. High doses of it have been found to aid in insulating nerve cells, increasing nerve conduction, and reducing the ear ringing associated with Bell's palsy. If you have an impeded facial movement on one side of the mouth, eating can be difficult, therefore soups or smoothies containing these types of nutrients are recommended. As an overall approach to your diet, reducing your intake of inflammatory foods is also suggested. For more details on anti-inflammatory diet options and a complete list of beneficial supplements turn, to Chapter 9.

Acupuncture can also help regenerate damaged nerves as it is thought to speed up muscle activity. Although there is no direct evidence of this, patient-based stories suggest that this therapy can aid in a rapid recovery.[14] To learn more about the healing benefits of acupuncture, turn to Chapter 8.

Cutting-edge therapies that are also useful in treating Bell's palsy include light-emitting diode therapy (LED) and pulsed electromagnetic-field therapy (PEMF). LED uses lights to penetrate the tissue and decrease inflammation, and PEMF utilizes electromagnetic pulses to reduce the pain associated with Bell's palsy. For more details on each of these therapies, refer to Chapters 11 and 12.

If there is permanent palsy damage to the face, then injections of botulinum toxin (Botox) or Dysport (an alternative to Botox), or even cosmetic surgery, which I like to call neuromodulators, can be used to restore symmetry to the face. The good news is that, in many cases, holistic and cutting-edge therapies help return the face to normal.

Rescued By Cutting-Edge Treatments

Lara, a fifty-nine-year-old Latin-American woman, came to see me after developing a facial paralysis related to Bell's palsy, and a subsequent outbreak of cold sores. In our meeting, she conveyed that she had been going through a stressful time before the onslaught of Bell's palsy. Her husband had been diagnosed with lung cancer, and soon after that her daughter had a miscarriage, followed by her ninety-one-year-old mother having a stroke and needing to be placed in a nursing home. During this time, Lara was depressed and exhausted, but she was so stressed out she couldn't sleep, which only worsened her already depleted state. For three months straight, Lara had painful headaches every single day. Then, one morning, she woke up unable to move her face. Lara's first thought was that, like her ninety-one-year-old mother, she was having a stroke. The paramedics rushed her to the emergency room where she was diagnosed with Bell's palsy and given prescription drugs of steroids and antivirals.

Three weeks later, when Lara came to my office, she had yet to see any improvement in her facial paralysis. I encouraged her by sharing my similar story of stress-induced Bell's palsy, and the treatments I had used to recover. I emphasized how vital it was to her regaining her health that she learn to reduce her stress through stress-management techniques. Lara took my treatment advice to heart and incorporated meditation and facial massage into her routine. She also began to consume foods that aided in healing her damaged nerves, and had acupuncture to help regenerate her nerves. Additionally, Lara took advantage of the cutting-edge therapies of LED and PEMF that I had discussed with her. Once her pain was under control, she added exercise and floating-tank therapy into her regimen to help manage her stress levels.

For Lara, it felt empowering to take active measures to heal, and those steps alone made her feel better about her situation. She found the floating-tank therapy truly relaxing and peaceful; it was during those sessions that she was able to forget the woes plaguing her family, finally stop crying, relax, and enter a meditative state. A few weeks after beginning the use of these alternative therapies, Lara felt happier and started to see improvement in her facial paralysis.

If you are experiencing stress-related Bell's palsy, a combination of holistic methods, cutting-edge treatments, and non-invasive procedures can work together to heal your symptoms.

PART TWO

Holistic Therapies

CHAPTERS 5–10

Chapters 5–10 examine how incorporating holistic measures, such as meditation, massages, acupuncture, breath and movement exercises, diet and supplements, even psychotherapy, into your lifestyle can help alleviate stress and heal skin and hair disorders.

5

Meditation

"Through meditation, you can calm the mind and develop what is important to you."

—YOGI BHAJAN

There was a time where every new year I found myself with the same resolution—to find more patience, balance, and peace in my life. It wasn't until I was in my forties that I began to search for a serious way to achieve this and discovered meditation. I started by simply setting aside five minutes of alone time every day (either morning or night) to relax and focus on my breathing. In 2006, I found the teachings of Tao and discovered how Taoist meditation could bring balance and harmony into my life.

Then, in 2008, a friend introduced me to transcendental meditation (TM), which provided me with the tools to meditate on a deeper level. After completing my training in transcendental meditation, whenever I felt stressed, I could go to my chosen quiet place and meditate for twenty minutes with TM techniques, after which I felt like a new person who could handle anything. This form of meditation is truly amazing—simple, effortless, and yet awe-inspiring. Despite the benefits I experienced using TM, I found it difficult to incorporate the recommended twenty minutes a day into my busy life as a single mom, physician, business owner, and caretaker for older parents, but when I was diagnosed with Bell's palsy in 2011, I realized that my health absolutely depended on my taking time out for meditation. Incorporating meditation into my life on a regular basis has had a tremendous impact on my sense of well-being and inner peace. I encourage you to explore the different types of meditation discussed in this chapter in order to experience the benefits for yourself.

So what is meditation, you may ask? The word *meditate* has its origins in the Latin word *meditatio* meaning to think, contemplate, devise, or ponder.[1] To meditate is to practice training your mind to be still, be in the present moment, and let your thoughts float by without attaching to them. By letting go of your thoughts and journeying within, a new awareness or consciousness can be created.

Almost all spiritual traditions practice meditation in some form, whether as the process of prayer, or looking within, or gathering light (as the Taoists believe). A codified practice of meditation evolved from the ancient Buddhist and Hindu religions. The scholar Richard Wilhelm is credited with introducing Eastern philosophies on meditation to the West in the early 1900s when he translated key Chinese texts into German that were subsequently translated into many other languages. Hindu meditation techniques also gained popularity in Western culture in the 1960s. It is important to note that you do not need to subscribe to a particular religious belief system to gain physical benefits from meditation. Taking time out from a hectic schedule to be present, to be silent, and to focus on positivity, has benefits for the body. Data has shown that meditating can serve to relax and reduce stress in the body, even though the exact mechanism of action (the way meditation physiologically acts on the body) remains unknown.[2] In my experience, meditation is a way to find inner peace, relaxation, calmness, happiness, and balance in the middle of a chaotic life. Practicing meditation allows you to detach from your problems, transcend stress, and find a way back to your core, your center.[3]

Meditation for Beginning Practitioners

A great way to start meditating is to simply set aside five minutes in the morning and evening to be alone with your thoughts, but, of course, if you can only start with once a day, it is better than nothing.

Pick a quiet place where you will not be interrupted, either by technological devices, family members, or cute pets that want your attention. Turn off all electronic equipment for those five minutes. Get in a comfortable position that is relaxed, but not lying down, as you want to avoid falling asleep. For that same reason, leave at least some light on in the room. To get positioned, close your eyes and breathe in deeply through your nose and out through your mouth. Really feel the breath as it leaves your throat. You may want to make a sound as you exhale. Focus only on your breathing. Anytime a disrupting sound or thought invades your quiet calmness, let it pass instead of latching onto it, and go back to your deep breathing. I like to use a timer to make sure I stay put for five minutes each time. If you are able to easily meditate for five minutes, then seek to increase your time to twenty minutes. The longer you meditate, the more your nervous system will have time to de-stress and the more benefits you will gain from this practice.

Meditation for Intermediate Practitioners

The book *Tao Te Ching* by Lao Tzu, which describes the Taoist philosophy of meditation, was written over twenty-five centuries ago and has been translated into more languages than any other book except the Bible. Tao means walking the path of wisdom; Te means virtue or good character; and Ching means a sacred book. This book is a spiritual guide that helps you create a path to peace within yourself, and find peace in the world around you. This type of meditation teaches people to observe their thoughts as they pass by, without attaching to them.

Diane Dreher's explanation of this philosophy in *The Tao of Inner Peace* is an easy read that describes the steps to follow in order to meditate, providing simple exercises, techniques, and daily affirmations. You can start at section one, with Taoist principles of balance and harmony, and progress slowly, or quickly, to section two where you integrate the principles of section one in order to bring peace into your life. From sections three, four, and five, you will learn to find both peace within and peace in the world around you.[4] There is no time limit for finishing the book, and you can return to different sections, as I did, learning something new each time. This is a great resource for anyone looking to advance to the next level of meditation, and find inner solace. Even as I progressed through the teachings of Tao, and completed the more advanced levels of meditation, I frequently went back to Dreher's book to re-read the meaningful affirmations and exercises. Life is a journey; stress can be either a bump or a giant rock in the road, and the teachings of Tao provide a path for you to move from imbalance and chaos to harmony and tranquility.

Meditation for Advanced Practitioners— Transcendental Meditation

While Taoist or Buddhist philosophies focus on observing thoughts during meditation and perfecting a concentrated, trained focus, transcendental meditation (TM) teaches the process of transcending your thoughts in order to access a deeper form of consciousness. TM teaches you not to fight with your thoughts to reach a meditative state, but to let go, and enter the transcended state with ease. TM techniques are best learned from an instructor. In order to explore this type of meditation, I recommend reading the autobiography of Paramahansa Yogananda, the first Yoga master of India, who published his book, *Autobiography of a Yogi,* in 1946. In it, he described his philosophy that started a spiritual revolution, especially in the West.[5]

So what exactly is TM? Well, you find a comfortable sitting position, and then recite a mantra or sound that is chosen for you by your TM instructor. As you breathe slowly, focusing on your mantra, muscles relax, and it is believed that prolactin (a hormone that appears to have a calming effect) is released. The purpose is to let your mind settle in the place beyond thought where the purest form of consciousness resides—the transcendental consciousness. This spiritual process provides participants with peace, harmony, and focus in their daily lives. It takes twenty minutes twice a day, and has such dramatic results that many who practice TM find, once they experience the benefits, they can't go without it. In fact, research confirms that brain activity connected to rest, reflection, focus, and competence is enhanced during TM.

Studies have shown TM works to treat many conditions, including high blood pressure, heart disease, attention deficit disorder, cancer, and, of course, stress.[6] Research conducted by the American Heart Association, American Psychological Association, National Institutes of Health, and the American Medical Association, all support the health benefits of transcendental meditation. In fact, a Stanford University study demonstrated that, compared to many other techniques, TM is twice as effective at reducing stress and anxiety.[7] Training in TM is offered in many areas, and certified teachers can be found online.

Restricted Environmental Stimulation Technique (Floatation REST)

This method of relaxation allows you to enter a meditative state by soaking in a tank filled with a high volume of Epsom salts, which serve to keep you afloat. The floating sensation and the silent environment in the tank facilitate the meditative process and allow stress to melt away. Generally, sessions in a floatation tank last sixty minutes, and the forced silence and solitude really do allow you to unwind in a quiet and calm environment without interruptions. This method of relaxation is proven to reduce stress-related pain,[8] as well as create an ideal environment for calming the mind and body. Initially used on animals and studied back in the 1980s, the benefits of this simple technique are not widely known.[9] The floating sensation creates an amazing and unusual experience; however, because the tank is a small, enclosed space, if you get claustrophobic, then this is probably not a good option for you.

So, whether you choose beginning, intermediate, or advanced meditation, make a concerted effort to commit to your health. Your body and mind will thank you for it. And when stress builds from a fight with your kids, a problem at work, or a disagreement with a friend, you will go to your place of peace, and be able to relax and find calm within yourself. After all, if you don't take the responsibility for creating balance in your life, who will?

6

Massages

"Too often we underestimate the power of a touch, a smile, a kind word, a listening ear, an honest compliment, or the smallest act of caring, all of which have the potential to turn a life around."

–LEO BUSCAGLIA

Ever wonder why the touch of someone's hand, a gentle caress, or a sturdy hug can give you goose bumps or make you feel warm all over? The healing power of touch is astounding. Massages have been shown to help relieve muscle aches and pains and also alleviate headaches, reduce tension and anxiety, and help with circulatory problems. Licensed massage therapists have become part of the mainstay of alternative medicine. Research demonstrates that massaging causes the body to release the endorphins serotonin and dopamine that calm the nervous system and lower the presence of the stress hormone, cortisol. Clinically, I have witnessed the healing effects of massages on my patients who have struggled with stress-induced illnesses, and in my own life, I have experienced how a massage can change the state of my being. Sixty minutes under the healing hands of a licensed masseur or masseuse has a long-lasting impact on my body, which is why I cherish my time on the massage table. In my experience, getting a massage on a weekly or semi-monthly basis is my secret for feeling a sense of calm as I go through my busy life. In fact, when I go too long without getting one, I can feel the tension mounting in my body. As the benefits of massage therapy have come to light, some companies are now offering it to their employees to help mitigate work-related stress.[1]

Massaging has the power to transport you from a chaotic state to a rested state. Have you ever passed by a person getting a massage in the mall? Amazingly, amid the hustle and bustle of shoppers, they are transported into a different world in the massage chair. Those minutes under the hands of a trained masseur or masseuse really can influence how the rest of your day proceeds. If you have ever had a massage, think how relaxed you felt when you got off the table to get dressed. In the warm afterglow, your body felt like mushy Jell-O, and you could barely walk straight. You felt euphoric, relaxed, peaceful, and perhaps a little groggy. You may have even felt healed from the stress or aches you came to the table with.

Several different types of massage therapy are described below. You may need to explore multiple types of massage before finding the technique that works best for your particular needs. Also, keep in mind that each massage therapist practices a bit differently, so it is important to find a therapist whose technique and touch elicit a good response in your body. And, always drink a large amount of water after each session, to rid your body of the toxins that were released during the massage.

TYPES OF MASSAGES

Swedish Massage

Swedish massage involves a gentle technique with long strokes and circular movements where the muscles are kneaded in order to relax and energize. There should be no discomfort with this form of massage.

Deep-Tissue Massage

As the title conveys, this is a form of massage that targets the deeper muscles in an effort to work out rooted knots, aches, and pains. This form of massage is usually performed on people with muscle aches and injuries, and firm pressure is used. Massage therapists will generally ask if they are using too much pressure, and you should always be vocal about what does and does not feel good (even if you are not asked).

Aromatherapy Massage

Essential oils, such as lavender, are used in conjunction with a massage to elicit a relaxing response while you are being worked on.

Shiatsu

This Japanese form of massages uses localized finger pressure along acupuncture meridians in a rhythmic sequence that works to massage the body and reduce stress.

Reflexology

Reflexology targets designated organ systems that are mapped out on the palm of your hand or the sole of your foot. Pressure is placed on these trigger points and that leads to a decrease in the discomfort of the related organs.

Thai Massage

In an effort to clear blocked energy, the technique of Thai massaging utilizes compression, pulling, and stretching, rather than kneading the muscles, to relieve tension. Therapists actually manipulate your body into yoga poses in order to stretch and elongate muscles, and to untwist or smooth out twisted or tightened internal organs.

Often, the healing effects of a massage are felt in your body for a few days, or even a week after the session. Soon though, life sets back in and the daily tasks and chores as parents, workers, bosses, students, and family members take over. Once again, you will need to find that time to relax, unwind, and heal. This is why it is important to incorporate an avenue of stress release into your life on a regular basis. Massages are a great way to relieve your body of harmful stress hormones, but this healing technique will have even better results for managing your stress when it's used in conjunction with exercise and meditation.[2]

7

Breath and Movement Techniques

"Happiness is when what you think, what you say, and what you do are in harmony."

—MAHATMA GANDHI

THE BENEFITS OF EXERCISE

Exercise is a vital tool for releasing stress from the body and it's important for your overall health. When stress builds up in the body, it can manifest as any one or more of a myriad of diseases, and can increase the risk of stress-induced skin and hair conditions, cardiovascular disease, and even cancer. Exercising on a regular basis can help reduce the likelihood of developing stress-induced diseases.[1]

For these reasons, one of the best things you can do for yourself is to incorporate some form of aerobic exercise (one that gets your heart rate elevated) into your routine. In addition to these benefits, exercise improves the way you feel and gives you energy. Over the last decade, studies have shown that aerobic exercise has antidepressant and anti-anxiety effects, which protect the body from the dangerous and harmful ramifications of stress.[2]

Given these obvious advantages, the question becomes, if exercise is incredibly beneficial and could literally save your life, why is it so hard to get out and do it? One reason could be, it can be overwhelming to figure out where to start, particularly if you haven't exercised in a long time, have never exercised on a regular basis, or have been dealing with a sickness or injury. When I'm trying to determine how to begin a momentous task, I say to myself, take it step by step. Surprisingly, these three little words can free you. Sometimes the overwhelming notion of getting in shape can make you feel pinned to your couch when what you really need to focus on instead is putting on your running shoes and walking out the front door and around the block. Or, you can aim so unrealistically high in your workout goals, like planning to run the LA Marathon when you haven't run in years, that you become overwhelmed by the notion. So, take it step-by-step. It's better to walk twenty minutes a day, three times a week, than set such lofty workout goals that you're rendered motionless. A consistent and modest workout on a regular basis is far better than a momentous workout on an infrequent basis.

When planning an exercise routine, it's also important to figure out what type of exercise you enjoy because the more you enjoy exercising, the more likely it is that you'll be motivated to go do it. If the gym feels like a torturous event, and you find yourself thinking you'd rather be at the dentist, then perhaps it's time to seek out a different type of exercise. Whether it's yoga, speed rope jumping (I'm fascinated with this now), boxing (I loved this until it hurt my knuckles to the point it was difficult to perform surgery), dancing (I still continue to do this for fun), the bar method, which is a mixture of ballet and yoga, or any other form of exercise available today, once you find a type you enjoy, you'll feel more motivated to work out. That's the great thing about exercise. Once your body begins to feel, and you begin to see, the positive effects of working out, your desire to exercise will grow. Therefore, as you gain momentum, the motivation and discipline to work out will become more automatic. Another tip for keeping motivated is to have a workout buddy. You two can schedule times to work out together and help push each other when one of you is feeling tired, or lazy, or depressed.

THE BENEFITS OF YOGA

> "Yoga is not a religion. It is a science, science of well-being, science of youthfulness, science of integrating body, mind and soul."
>
> –AMIT RAY, *YOGA AND VIPASSANA: AN INTEGRATED LIFE STYLE*

Yoga—meaning to unite body, mind, and soul—is a five-thousand-year-old practice. It combines postures (asanas), chanting, and deep-breathing (pranayama) activities with exercise poses that strengthen the body's core and flexibility. For our purposes here, there are also stress-reducing benefits that come from practicing this form of exercise. Yoga incorporates meditation with movement, and this has a centering effect. The deep breathing and the postures of yoga cultivate an awareness of the body and help practitioners journey inward to discover both the physical and emotional state of their body. Many of my patients who do yoga report that they feel less stress and an overall sense of peace and well-being from this practice.

Studies have shown that the deep breathing utilized when practicing yoga leads to the relaxation response and lessens muscle tension, both of which serve to reduce the presence of stress hormones.[3] In fact, a study conducted on first-year medical students found that yoga had anxiety-reducing effects on those students who practiced it regularly. Even during their exceedingly stressful exam time, the medical students who practiced yoga were able to reduce the anxiety surrounding the high-pressure situation. Interestingly—in the yoga control group, more medical students passed the exam than did medical students who were *not* practicing yoga. If yoga could serve to mitigate the stress of medical students during exams, it could certainly serve to reduce your stress and anxiety when you, too, face high-pressure situations in your life. This study also found that, in addition to reducing stress, the students who practiced yoga also reported a "better sense of well-being, feelings of relaxation, improved concentration, self-confidence, improved efficiency, good interpersonal relationships, increased attentiveness, lowered irritability levels, and an optimistic outlook on life."[4] Now, those are all amazing benefits from a form of exercise.

In order to get these benefits, you will have to venture out and try this exercise routine. You can begin with a DVD at home. One of my patients, Kimberly Fowler, a survivor and an inspiration, has an excellent line of yoga videos called *Yoga for Athletes.* For more details on her videos, you can turn to the Resources section in the back of the book. Taking yoga classes at your local gym is also an option. For the authentic yoga experience, you will need a warm quiet room and a purposefully guided practice. You should visit a yoga studio because oftentimes yoga classes at the gym are loud and not long enough to really get a good workout.

There are numerous forms of yoga, and most yoga studios subscribe to a particular type of practice. Examples of the various types of yoga practices include Vinyasa, Purna, Ashtanga, Jnana, Bhakti, Bikram, Karma, Raja, Hatha, Kundalini, Mantra, Tantra, Iyengar, Vini, Ananda, Anusara, Integral, Kali Ray Tri, Kripalu, and Sivananda, to name a few. The most popular forms of yoga are listed below.

Hatha Yoga

This ancient form of yoga combines breath and postures with the goal of aligning energy and providing purification. It includes slow smooth movements, holding poses, and concentrating on breathing. Good for beginners, to stretch, relax, and decrease stress. Many other forms of Western yoga have evolved from the practice of Hatha yoga.

Ashtanga Vinyasa

This form of yoga combines breath work and movement through posture sequences meant to guide the practitioner through a moving meditation. Beginning classes move slowly through the postures while more advanced classes move rapidly through postures, which are designed to build heat in the body.

Bikram

Bikram yoga consists of twenty-six postures taken from the Hatha yoga process, that are practiced in an extremely hot room (temperatures can reach up to 105 degrees). The poses are stationary and repetitive and presented in the exact same order every class. Those who enjoy static poses tend to prefer Bikram, while those who enjoy moving through a variety of poses, tend to prefer Vinyasa. This type of yoga is great for sweating out toxins and loosening tight muscles, which helps with chronic pain; practitioners should be aware, however, that there is a risk of dehydration.

Overall, keep in mind that making exercise part of your weekly routine will benefit your body and mind, uplift your spirit, and reduce your stress levels. A healthy lifestyle starts with one step. Once you take enough steps toward a healthy lifestyle, and find a form of exercise you really enjoy doing, then exercise will be a regular part of your life, and you will have more energy, and feel more positive about life.

8

Acupuncture

> "There is nothing that can be said so certainly about stress except that the amount of rest produced will neutralize the corresponding intensity of stress."
>
> —MAHARISHI MAHESH YOGI

Acupuncture originated in ancient China around 100 BC. The roots of this healing technique are tied to the Taoist philosophy mentioned in the chapter on meditation. According to the discourse governing this therapeutic technique, the body contains two types of energy: yin and yang. When these energies are flowing properly, the body is balanced and healthy. When the energy gets blocked, illness occurs. Acupuncture clears blocked energy and, in so doing, restores the body's balance.[1]

In China, acupuncture was used in conjunction with herbs, massage, heat, and diet. The first book explaining the theory of acupuncture, *The Great Compendium of Acupuncture and Moxibustion (Heat*), was published in the fourteenth century during the Ming Dynasty. This book described the three hundred and sixty-five needle-insertion points that are believed to modify the flow of qi, or energy. At first, because Western medicine was unable to quantify how acupuncture works, it viewed this therapeutic technique with skepticism. In the 1950s, however, this began to change with Professor Ji-Sheng Han's dramatic research at the Neurological Institute, Peking University, demonstrating that acupuncture triggered a physiological response in the body with the release of neurotransmitters and opioid peptides. As a result, the use of acupuncture as a medical treatment began to spread. In the 1970s, a team of U.S. physicians headed to China to find out more about this technique, opening the door to this treatment that was gaining popularity in the West. While the exact mechanisms of action (the way acupuncture works) still remain unverified, studies do show that acupuncture has healing benefits.

Research data from the National Institutes of Health shows that acupuncture needles stimulate nerve endings and alter brain function, thereby proving that acupuncture does work on the neuroendocrine immune system and does inhibit pain. Acupuncture also functions to decrease the heart rate and lower blood pressure, and can serve to relax muscles, all of which reduce stress in the body. According to the Eastern philosophy of acupuncture, stress is believed to block the free flow of energy (qi). Acupuncture operates to facilitate the flow of energy by clearing blocks and allowing it to flow smoothly, which, in turn, minimizes stress and the symptoms of stress. Typically, needles are used, but beads, ultrasound, or physical manipulation with hands (acupressure) are also used. These are placed along meridian lines, which are thought to be the pathways of energy. When there is an imbalance, the acupuncture points along these meridian lines become red or tender. The Chinese word for meridian is *ching-lo,* which means to pass through and connect, respectively. There are twelve meridians, referred to as the major trunks, which are the connecting pathways to the organ for which they are named. The placement of needles or pressure on the meridians creates a flow of energy between meridians. Scientifically, meridians can be seen on infrared imaging as they appear to possibly be polarized, stable water clusters.[2]

Whether acupuncture works by balancing the flow of energy (the life force called qi), or by stimulating nerves, muscles, and connective tissue at points of needle insertion, acupuncture appears to increase the blood flow. This increase in the flow of blood to cells serves to clear out cortisol and other stress hormones, and increase the release of endorphins, the body's natural form of painkillers.[3] To this end, a Georgetown study demonstrated that acupuncture lowered stress in animal models.[4]

When I had a partial facial paralysis due to Bell's palsy, I was willing to try any type of treatment. A patient of mine, an ophthalmologist who had also experienced Bell's palsy, relayed to me that acupuncture had sped up her recovery. Even though I didn't like the idea of having needles in my face, a speeded-up recovery certainly sounded good, so I went for it and sat patiently as the needles and an electromagnetic machine were attached to the palsied side of my face. When the machine contracted, so did my paralyzed muscles. I continued my treatments twice a week until my palsy started to resolve at week three, and I regained movement in my face. While I can't know for sure if acupuncture was responsible for my recovery, I did feel as though the muscles in my face were being stimulated during treatments. And the data I read on the healing effects of acupuncture was quite convincing.[5]

Several different types of acupuncture are described below, so you can choose the type of treatment that feels right for you.

TYPES OF ACUPUNCTURE

Meridian Therapy—Japanese-Style Acupuncture

This technique uses thin needles or moxa (moxibustion, which is burning mugwort applied to the skin to create a warm sensation) to apply pressure along meridian locations, or energy pathways. In the areas of needle insertion, electromagnetic energy is released through small electrical charges to regenerate nerves and alter neurotransmitters. This is the type of acupuncture I utilized to aid in my recovery from Bell's palsy. During this form of acupuncture, the electromagnetic energy can be a little unnerving, but otherwise the treatment generally relaxes the person being treated into a meditative state.[6]

Auricular Acupuncture

This type of acupuncture operates under the theory that the ear is a microsystem representing the entire body. Auricular (ear) models demonstrate acupuncture points that affect all parts of the body, and indicate where the needle placement for each condition is needed. After needles are placed in ear points, you can have acupuncture beads placed in special locations along the ear that are specifically designed to relieve stress. Then, anytime during the day or night, you can press the beads to relieve stress. Controversial data suggests that auricular acupuncture may also reduce appetite and help with fertility. The beads can stay on for about 2–4 days.[7] This is a popular technique used by many celebrities.

Traditional Chinese Medicine (TCM) Acupuncture

Acupuncturists use eight principles of complementary opposites (yin/yang, internal/external, excess/deficiency, hot/cold) to treat imbalances in the body and the resulting conditions, in an effort to return harmony to the body. These principles are evaluated on a case-by-case basis, so the cause of an imbalance determines the combination of therapies used. This form of acupuncture combines a mixture of adjunctive therapies, such as acupressure, heat, massage, meditation, herbal medicine, and exercise.[8]

French Energetic Acupuncture

Physicians generally perform this mixed-style acupuncture where needles are placed in key areas based on the principles of neuroanatomy. Needles are inserted at meridian points according to the principles of a yin and yang energy flow. Yin energy flows upward toward heaven, and yang energy flows downward toward earth.[9]

Korean Hand Acupuncture

Developed in 1971 by Dr. Tae Woo Yoo, this technique uses reflexology and acupressure to apply pressure to particular points in the hands and feet that are believed to affect a corresponding body part. Treatments can also include taped-on metal acupressure pellets and infrared heat, miniature acupuncture needles, and electrical stimulation. Similar to auricular acupuncture, hands and feet are believed to represent the body as a whole.[10]

Myofascially-Based Acupuncture

Myofascial trigger points were discovered in the 1800s, and they appear to be quite similar to acupuncture points. Therapists feel along meridian lines looking for tender points and place needles at the sites of an abnormal energy flow. Using acupuncture in combination with myofascial trigger positions reduces pain and swelling by accessing muscle trigger points. Often, deep-pressure massage, mechanical vibration, and electrical stimulation are incorporated into myofascial trigger-point therapy.[11]

Sonopuncture

Also known as vibrational medicine, acutonics uses an ultrasonic device instead of needle acupuncture to send sound waves to points in the body. Crafted tuning forks, chimes, Tibetan bowls, and musical instruments are placed at acupoints to stimulate an individual's energy fields.[12]

Acupressure

This healing technique uses hands, fingers, palms, elbows, or feet in place of needles to put pressure on energy pathways in the body and relieve pain. The Japanese form of acupressure is known as shiatsu, which employs the same energy meridians or acupoints as acupuncture. Stretching can be added to an acupressure massage to create balance.[13]

Whatever form of acupuncture therapy you decide to use, this healing therapy can help manage stress, relieve pain, and aid you in your journey to health. It's important to drink a lot of water after undergoing an acupuncture session because once your blocked energy is cleared, toxins are released into the body, and water is needed to flush the toxins out.

This healing technique is best used in conjunction with the other holistic methods of stress management discussed in Part Two.

9

Diet and Supplements

> "It is health that is real wealth and not pieces of gold and silver."
>
> –MAHATMA GANDHI

Diet

The foods you consume play a crucial role in the health of your skin and hair. Stress has harmful effects on both of these, ranging from aging to rashes to rosacea to hair loss,[1] and your diet is a powerful tool that can be wielded to combat these negative effects. If you choose badly, your daily meals can worsen the effects of stress in your body, but if you choose wisely, your nutritional choices can help you reduce the effects of stress in your body.

Stress increases the levels of the hormone cortisol, which is in the glucocorticoid family. Cortisol in your body raises blood sugar (glucose), increases blood pressure, damages the immune system, and incites inflammation, which thins out and ages your skin and hair. When stress increases your cortisol levels, it is important to balance the stress hormones in your system and calm your daily existence by filling your body with nutrition that lowers blood sugar, levels blood pressure, and reduces inflammation.

What is the key to a stress-busting diet?… consuming foods that reduce inflammation, and avoiding foods that trigger inflammation and cause a host of skin and hair conditions. To keep the inflammation down, I follow the golden rule I learned through the "Growing Great Nutrition Program" at my son and daughter's elementary school, which champions eating foods that are "whole, close to the source, and minimally processed."

This concept is simple enough that even an eight-year-old can follow it, and it's one I not only reinforce with my children, but teach to my patients, as well. Here are some recommendations along these lines.

- Pay attention to the list of ingredients on package labels, being careful to avoid processed foods.
- Avoid saturated fats and processed carbohydrates.
- Eat good fats, such as the mono- or polyunsaturated fats found in avocados, olives and olive oil, tofu nuts, and fatty fish.
- Coconut oil is a healthy unsaturated fat that can be used to cook just about anything.
- Seek out colorful fruits and vegetables, and unprocessed carbohydrates (whole wheat products, including flour, brown rice, etc.).
- Beans, especially lentils (my daughter loves my lentil soup), are a great carbohydrate option.
- When consuming protein, seek out grass-fed beef, or natural, antibiotic-free chicken.
- Wild salmon is also an excellent protein option and, if you marinate it in low-sodium soy sauce as I do for my children, they will not complain that it tastes fishy. Or, after marinating it, sprinkling it with fresh lemon juice, salt, cayenne pepper, and dillweed is another great way to prepare it.

THREE NUTRITIONAL PLANS

In the following section, I am providing summaries of three nutritional plans touted by doctors and specialists to keep inflammation down. These approaches provide variations on the theme of eating whole, close to the source, and minimally processed. While I do not necessarily believe in every detail of the diets discussed below, I do believe they are a good start for reducing the consumption of foods that can worsen stress and lead to consequential disease states. It's not about following a diet in a strict and rigid manner, it can be unhealthy to become obsessed with following a stringent regimen. Instead, try to make healthy choices eighty percent of the time, and look for nutritional choices that make you feel and look better. You may decide to pick and choose elements from each nutritional plan that work for you. I definitely like to mix and match my meal choices. Or, you may choose to seek the advice of a healthcare professional involved in nutrition and alternative medicine. Above all, refer back to this mantra… *keep it whole, close to the source, and minimally processed.* To learn more about each of these nutritional programs, I have attached references.

Dr. Floyd H. Chilton

Dr. Floyd H. Chilton's book, *Win the War Within: The Eating Plan That's Clinically Proven to Fight Inflammation—The Hidden Cause of Weight Gain and Chronic Disease,* approaches nutrition from an anti-inflammatory angle. He believes that, to help prevent disease states, you must fight to reduce or prevent inflammation in your body. Dr. Chilton's premise is to reduce inflammation before it starts, if possible, and bring down the building blocks of inflammation messengers.

His program reduces omega-6 fatty acid (specifically arachidonic acid), high glycemic-index foods, especially high glycemic-index carbohydrates, and pro-inflammatory foods, such as egg yolks, and replaces them with non-starchy vegetables (kale, broccoli, spinach, mushrooms, tomatoes, asparagus, squash), nuts and seeds, wild/grass fed/organic lean protein (beef, pork, shellfish, fatty fish). Cooking with olive oil or coconut oil affords healthier fatty acids. Simply stated, Chilton's program focuses on whole foods, nutrient-dense carbohydrates, lean proteins, and beneficial fatty acids. The Inflammatory Index of chapter 13 in Chilton's book makes it easy to see how many inflammatory foods are in your diet, and helps you know the worse offenders, followed with a short list of glycemic-index levels and examples.[2]

Here is a quick daily meal plan based on Chilton's theories.[3]

Breakfast	$^1/_2$ cup nonfat cottage cheese or nonfat Greek yogurt, $^1/_4$ cup fresh blueberries, $^1/_2$ cup oatmeal
Lunch	4–6 ounce flank steak with orange vinaigrette over spinach, fresh grapes
Dinner	4–6 jumbo shrimp and vegetable stir-fry in olive oil, with whole-wheat tortilla, brown rice
Snack	One small apple, sliced, with almond butter, or $^1/_2$ cup roasted nuts

Dr. Nicholas Perricone

In his book, *The Perricone Promise: Look Younger Live Longer in Three Easy Steps,* Dr. Nicholas Perricone proposes a three-step approach to decreasing inflammation on a cellular level. His premise is that stress increases your "death hormones" (cortisol and insulin), which damage your body by increasing inflammation. The inflammation created by the food you put in your body can be just as harmful as the inflammation created by stress, or *death* hormones, as they both cause your skin and organs to age. The end game: decrease inflammation, and thereby decrease stress and aging.[4]

He proposes that you increase the consumption of peptides and neuropeptides, which can repair scars, aid in the production of collagen and elastin, and speed up wound repair. These elements also elevate the efficiency of your metabolism, which leads to such additional benefits as cellular repair, mood elevation, and immune-system rejuvenation. Consuming these elements can also lead to denser bones, a healthier heart, and a decreased risk of certain cancers.[5] Dr. Perricone's nutritional regimen follows the same mantra I learned from my daughter's third grade nutrition teachers. "Buy your foods in their most natural, unprocessed state," then "add your own fresh or dried herbs and spices." Overall, employing the nutritional approach he suggests will help you look and feel younger and will serve to reduce inflammation, which will assist in combating the stress-induced skin and hair conditions discussed in this book. Dr. Perricone recommends the foods outlined below that are packed full of beneficial peptides and neuropeptides.

- **Carotenoids** (carrots, wild Alaskan salmon, shellfish, kale, spinach, colorful fruits and vegetables, pomegranates). Antioxidant, reduces pain and inflammation.
- **Limonoids and limonenes** (citrus fruits). These detoxify the liver, lower cholesterol, and inhibit cancer in lab animals.
- **Flavonoids** (non-carotenoid antioxidants in fruits and vegetables, blueberries). These fight free radicals and inflammation, inhibit cancer growth, protect blood vessels, and neutralize infection.
- **Flavon-3-ols** (acai, white/green/ black tea, grapeseed extract, pycnogenol). These antioxidants neutralize free radicals, inhibit tumor growth, and rectify bad cholesterol levels.
- **Glucosinolates and indoles** (cruciferous vegetables, such as broccoli, kale, Brussels sprouts). These are super antioxidants that have anticancer properties and help estrogen metabolism.

If nothing else from this diet excites you, at least add the following 10 superfoods Dr. Perricone mentions, which, consistent with my research, point to better, healthier living.

1. Acai fruit, in juice form or in smoothies
2. Garlic, leeks, shallots
3. Barley
4. Blue-green algae or wheat grass
5. Buckwheat
6. Beans and lentils
7. Hot peppers
8. Nuts and seeds
9. Sprouts
10. Yogurt and kefir

Below are a few meal suggestions based on Perricone's theories.

Breakfast	Turkey bacon, 1/2 cup nonfat cottage cheese, 1/2 cup buckwheat cereal, one kiwi, 8 ounces green tea or filtered water
Snack	Plain yogurt mixed with acai berry or powder, 3 walnuts, and 8 ounces of filtered water
Lunch	1/2 cup hummus, 4–6 ounces broiled wild salmon, 2 celery stalks, and one apple
Snack	1–2 ounces of chicken breast, 1/4 cup pumpkin seeds, 1/2 cup cherries, 8 ounces of filtered water
Dinner	Grilled Indian chicken, 1/2 cup baked barley, 2-inch cantaloupe wedge, and 8-ounces of filtered water[6]

Gluten-Free Diet

Gluten-free diets can help reduce inflammation and are beneficial for women who are pre-menopausal or going through menopause, as studies have found that avoiding gluten products can help minimize the symptoms of menopause. Gluten is a protein complex found in products containing wheat, flour, barley, rye, and triticale (a hybrid between rye and wheat). This diet is vital for individuals with celiac disease, who are intolerant of the gluten protein, due to damage in the small intestine's digestion process. Oats have been declared gluten-free recently, however, many celiacs continue to have mild to severe reactions to them.

For women going through menopause, this diet is helpful. Studies have linked menopausal symptoms to the gluten protein, and women on gluten-free diets appear to have much lighter menopausal symptoms. Gluten-free diets have led to less painful menses and a delayed menopause, as well as decreases in headaches, joint aches, and mood changes. There is a distinct connection between gluten sensitivity and low ovarian reserve.[7] For this reason, women with low levels of estradiol (a sex hormone) who are under the age of forty should consider cutting gluten from their diet. And for women concerned about the symptoms of menopause (a family history of a difficult transition through menopause tends to run in families), choosing a gluten-free diet may be warranted.

Right now, there are many gluten-free products and menu options in restaurants that make this diet simpler than before. This type of nutritional plan focuses on eating fruits, vegetables, and lean protein with gluten-free carbohydrates, such as brown rice and quinoa. In order to eliminate gluten from your diet, you have to become a gluten detective. Besides avoiding obvious gluten-based foods, such as breads, pastries, pastas, baked goods, gravies, soups, sauces, and casseroles (unless you have verified they do not contain gluten), you need to know the secret names given to gluten. Labels do not generally state gluten as an ingredient, so you have to know the names of ingredients frequently used for thickening or flavoring that may be derived from a gluten grain. Some of these ingredients include hydrolyzed vegetable protein, autolyzed yeast, soy sauce, caramel color, and starch, to name a few. It may be hard to believe, but if you are consuming BBQ'd potato chips, Chinese food, beer, cola, or just some clear, canned chicken broth, you are probably getting a good dose of gluten.

If you have a craving for baked goodies, gluten-free breads, brownies, cookies, and other treats can be found at an increasing number of stores, including Whole Foods and other health food stores. I have found that the easiest gluten-free nutrition plan to incorporate in daily life is Tammi Credicott's book *The Healthy Gluten-Free Life: 200 Delicious Gluten-Free, Dairy-Free, Soy-Free, and Egg-Free Recipes.*[8]

The monthly magazine, *Gluten-Free Living,* also has delicious recipes that make living gluten-free tastier than ever. Here is an example of a daily meal plan.

Breakfast	Sweet potato hash with eggs
Snack	1 piece of fruit and Indian spiced cashews
Lunch	Asian bean salad with tahini dressing
Snack	Roasted tomato and garlic spread
Dinner	Grilled shrimp brochettes and quinoa timbales with roasted peppers and herbs

The American Academy of Dermatology has even come up with a list of food and drink that can prematurely age your skin; it includes sweets, alcohol, white wine, charred meat, salty foods, and processed meats.

Supplements

In a perfect world, you would get all the nutrients and supplements you need through your diet. But as you age, your nutritional requirements shift, and, of course, individual needs vary based on family history, genetics, lifestyle, and a myriad of other factors. There are thousands of supplements, ranging from vitamins and minerals to herbal preparations, and other natural ingredients. My recommendations, outlined below, are based on my research and focus on what I believe to be the most beneficial supplements for the stress-related skin and hair conditions described in this book. While the following supplements are not a substitute for the good health and nutrition described in the first part of this chapter, they are meant to work as a complement to your healthy eating. When purchasing supplements, it's important to seek out "respected manufacturers with good manufacturing practices."[9] Reading reviews of supplement brands online is a good place to start. Also, since there can be drug interactions with some supplements, prior to taking any, it's important to review details of the supplements and their possible complications. Discussing them with an informed physician or alternative medicine doctor is important, too, as the suggested dosage of each supplement varies based on individual needs. Most nutrition books, including the books mentioned above by Chilton and Perricone, currently combine the use of supplements in their recommendations.

HERE ARE THE SUPPLEMENTS I RECOMMEND

Vitamins

They are essential for normal cell functions and work in conjunction with minerals as components of enzymes and coenzymes that carry out important chemical processes in the body. To find out the appropriate doses for each, discuss them with your nutritionist or doctor.

- **Beta-carotene** (fat-soluble). This is an antioxidant converted to vitamin A. It helps to prevent cancer and works as an immune enhancer.

  Best found in bright orange-colored fruits and vegetables (carrots, apricots, yams, squash) and red and purple fruits and vegetables (red cabbage, berries, and plums)

- **Carotenoids.** The carotenoid astaxanthin is an organic pigment with a high antioxidant level that is found in the fruits and vegetables listed above, and in dark leafy greens, wild salmon, trout, and shrimp.

- **B-Complex.** This water-soluble vitamin supports the immune system.

  Vitamin B_2 (riboflavin). This is part of two enzymes involved in the production of energy by converting food (carbohydrates) into fuel (glucose), which is then burned by the body to produce energy. Studies have shown this vitamin can reduce the frequency and severity of headaches, and migraines.

  Vitamin B_6 (pyridoxine). Helps in the production of protein as a necessary cofactor in the formation of enzymes for stress. It works to maintain proper immune function, stabilize hormones, and reduce migraine severity. Low levels of this vitamin are found in people with depression.

  Vitamin B_{12} (cobalamin). In addition to DNA synthesis, this vitamin helps with the insulation surrounding nerve cells, which increases nerve conduction, reduces the ear ringing (tinnitus) of Bell's palsy, as well as the eye-twitching seen in stress. It also helps with the exhaustion associated with herpes zoster (shingles) and to reset the circadian rhythm that is disrupted by stress. This vitamin is found in liver, kidney, eggs, fish, cheese, and meat. People who are depressed, or older people with impaired mental function, and those with multiple sclerosis, have been found to have low levels of this vitamin.

- **Vitamin C** (water-soluble). This vitamin acts as an antioxidant, stimulates collagen production, and helps with wound healing. It improves immune function, as well as the transmission of nerve-impulse substances, such as carnitine, tyrosine, neurotransmitters, and hormones/steroids. For these reasons, this vitamin helps treat eruptions of the herpes zoster virus (shingles). Vitamin C helps to support adrenal function and decrease elevated cortisol levels. It also reduces the risk of all forms of cancer, prevents the secretion of histamines by white blood cells, and increases the breakdown of histamines. This helps with asthma and allergies. During times of stress and/or infection, much higher doses are needed.
- **Vitamin D** (fat-soluble). Helps with calcium absorption and is necessary for bone stability.
- **Vitamin E** (fat-soluble). This is mainly an antioxidant that protects against cell-membrane damage and supports and improves the immune system. For this reason, it helps treat the virus herpes zoster (shingles). It is associated with preventing cancer, and also works to moisturize the skin, and improve menopausal symptoms.
- **Women's vitamin combinations** that contain phytoestrogens (plant-derived estrogen-like chemicals). These serve to counterbalance the increase of male hormone production.

Minerals

Essential minerals are necessary for normal cell function and work in conjunction with vitamins as components of enzymes and coenzymes that carry out important chemical processes in the body.

- **Calcium.** This acts as building blocks for bones and teeth, as an anti-inflammatory, and as an aid in muscle contraction. It also has a role in the release of neurotransmitters and relaxes the nervous system. This mineral assists in blood clotting, preventing colon cancer, and boosting energy. Consumption of calcium needs to be combined with magnesium for appropriate absorption.

- **Copper.** Helps to heal wounds, prevent wrinkles, and fight against heart disease and acne.

  Copper is naturally found in meats, poultry, eggs, nuts, seeds, and grains. Multivitamins often contain enough copper to supplement the amount you consume from your diet.

- **Iron.** Involved in energy production, metabolism, and DNA synthesis. It also serves to transport oxygen.

  This mineral is naturally found in leafy greens and grass-fed beef.

- **Magnesium.** Low amounts of this mineral lead to stress, insomnia, and PMS. Activates enzymes to reduce migraine pain, and reduces stress and fatigue. The combination of calcium/magnesium serves to relax the nervous system, and helps with cardiac disorders and attention deficit disorder. These two minerals taken in tandem also boost energy and act as anti-inflammatories.

- **Selenium.** This is one of the strongest antioxidants. It attacks free radicals, reduces an overactive immune system, and improves moods. Anecdotal evidence shows it works to reduce inflammatory conditions, such as eczema and psoriasis.[9] It is also useful in treating eruptions of the herpes zoster virus (shingles).

- **Zinc.** This mineral is essential for immune function, wound healing, and skin health. It helps treat the herpes zoster virus (shingles), improves acne, and is necessary for the function of hormones, such as: growth hormones, sex hormones, and insulin.

Herbs

- **Curcumin.** Antimicrobial, antioxidant, anti-inflammatory, and anti-cancer properties are seen. However, oral absorption is difficult, and topically the bright yellow color is a deterrent. More studies are working on increasing the utility of this spice.[10]
  From turmeric (the main ingredient of curry powder).

- **Feverfew.** This inhibits inflammatory substances, histamine release, and blood-vessel-dilating substances (histamine and serotonin). It also relieves migraines and rheumatoid arthritis.
  Found in sunflowers.

- **Ginger.** This important herb inhibits inflammation, lowers cholesterol, and improves migraines and motion sickness. It also acts as an antioxidant and helps to reduce nausea.

- **Lavender oil.** This has relaxing properties and acts as an antioxidant.

- **Milk thistle.** This contains silymarin, an antioxidant and detoxifying flavonoid, which inhibits inflammatory compounds. This serves to reduce the stimulation of plaque formation in psoriasis. This substance also protects the liver and restores liver cells.

- **Oil of oregano.** This has antibacterial properties.

- **Polypodium leucotomos.** This is a species of fern from South America that is made into a supplement for sun protection. It acts as an antioxidant to fight free radicals. Can be found over the counter in the antioxidant formula, Heliocare, and should be taken daily.[12]

- **Valerian.** Attaches to brain receptors and is used as a sedative for insomnia, anxiety, and stress.

Natural Ingredients

- **Y-Linolenic acid** (omega-6 fatty acid). This acid reduces the severity of eczema, and reduces allergies, blood pressure, and cholesterol. This acid also boosts the metabolism of fat and energy.
  Found in blue green algae, and spirulina.

- **Acetyl-L-carnitine.** Acts as an antioxidant, boosts energy, and metabolizes fat. Also involved in blocking substance P (which causes aging). Protects the nervous system, and restores brain cells and cortisol receptors, which protect nerve cells from stress.
  Found in beef, chicken, and pork.

- **Alpha-lipoic acid.** This acid acts as an antioxidant, has anti-aging effects, boosts energy, and metabolizes fat. It is also involved in preventing and repairing collagen damage. It also prevents accumulation of stress proteins in heart tissue following stress and increases their elimination.[13]

- **Amino acids** (arginine, cysteine, lysine, and methionine). These are essential for making proteins in the skin, such as collagen and elastin. These amino acids have antiviral effects and are useful in treating eruptions of the virus herpes zoster (shingles). They are also necessary for enzyme production and the transport of iron, and they serve to improve the liver's ability to remove excess toxins and hormones from the body.
  Found in high-protein meat, poultry, eggs, fish (cod and sardines), and vegetables.

- **Bee Power** (royal jelly extract). This extract fights free radicals, acts as an anti-inflammatory, reduces infections, and helps stop the growth of cancer.

- **CoQ_{10}.** Decreases substance P, which has aging effects, helps reduce the effects of migraines, and boosts the metabolism of fat and energy. Also acts as an antioxidant and anti-inflammatory. It reduces free radicals and has potential anticancer properties.

- **Flaxseed oil** or fresh crushed flaxseed. This is rich in omega-3 fatty acids. It contains a class of phytoestrogens (plant-derived estrogen-like chemicals). Also acts as an antioxidant and anti-inflammatory. Controls blood sugar and insulin, reduces the risk of diabetes, hormone-related cancers, and cardiovascular disease. Flaxseed is known to improve gastrointestinal health.
- **Gamma linolenic acid** (omega-6 fatty acid). Reduces the severity of eczema, as well as allergies, blood pressure, and cholesterol levels. Boosts the metabolism of fat and energy.

  Found in blue-green algae and spirulina.
- **Glucosamine** (amino monosaccharides). Acts as a skin lightener, but also increases production of hyaluronic acid in skin and joints. This supplement repaired sun damage in mice and has anti-inflammatory activities.[14,15]
- **Glycyrrhetinic acid.** This licorice extract has similar effects to topical hydrocortisone and acts as an anti-inflammatory.
- **Hops** (like those used to brew beer). These help with anxiety and sleeplessness.
- **Lecithin** (a natural by-product of the liver). Cleanses the liver and removes fatty liver deposits.
- **Maca.** Lowers menopausal symptoms and anxiety.
- **Primrose oil.** This contains omega-6 essential fatty acids and inhibits the conversion of testosterone to dihydrotestosterone, which causes hair loss. It also contains gamma linoleic acid that helps treat inflammatory skin conditions and cancer.
- **Omega-3 essential fatty acids.** Containing DHA and EPA, this reduces the signs and symptoms of allergies and inflammation. It boosts energy and brain and heart health.

- **Docosohexaenoic acid (DHA).** This inhibits 5-alpha reductase, the enzyme that converts testosterone into DHT (causing more hair growth).

  Found in salmon, sardines, and tuna.

- **Quercetin.** A bioflavonoid with anti-inflammatory and anti-allergy properties. Also acts as an antioxidant. Shown to inhibit the manufacture and release of histamine and inflammatory mediators, and prevent cancer and infections.

  Found in onions.

- **S-adenosylmethionine.** This increases brain chemicals, such as serotonin, dopamine, and phosphatidylserine.[16]

- **Serenoa repens** (saw palmetto fan palm). This extract reduces oily skin and excess hair growth.

  Saw-palmetto-berry extract is derived from the deep purple berries of the above-listed palm tree

- **Prebiotics and black currant-seed oil.** This contains essential fatty acids—specifically all three forms of linolenic acid. Reduces the development of AD (atopic dermatitis, eczema).[17]

- **Probiotics** (*Lactobacillus rhamnosus* GG). These are healthy intestinal bacteria that appear to prevent atopic dermatitis (eczema)[18] and asthma by affecting the body's nutritional status and immune-system functioning. They also reduce inflammatory disease, especially of the intestines, as well as the risk of cardiovascular disease or cancer.

  Found in yogurt and kefir.

- **Pycnogenol** (a flavon-3-ol). Acts as an antioxidant and an anti-inflammatory. It also prevents infection, helps to prevent cancer, and improves heart health.

  Found in pine bark extract.

- **Viviscal.** This is an all-natural supplement made from deep-sea fish protein, trademarked *aminomar C.* A Scandinavian professor discovered this ingredient while studying the source of the luscious hair and beautiful skin of the Inuit population. The supplement was invented in 1980 and has been utilized in the modeling world for decades. My office has performed numerous studies examining the effects of Viviscal on nail and hair growth and has had amazing results.[19] The biggest complaint I hear from my women patients is that their hair grows so fast they have to color it more frequently. This supplement is useful for both men and women who are experiencing hair loss due to stress and aging, as well as for other hair-loss conditions.

For more details about the supplements that are right for you, see your health specialist. There are many other natural, non-prescription health remedies available. Above all, be fully aware that your diet-supplement routine can have a huge effect on your health.

In addition to a healthy diet, I take supplements on a regular basis, as do my kids, and we are rarely sick, so I think there is merit to incorporating supplements in your diet. My grandfather also routinely took supplements, in addition to a healthy diet, and he was the healthiest man I knew. He became a vegetarian at the age of seventeen and every day he ate raw garlic (he certainly smelled like it), which reduces high blood pressure and high cholesterol and is thought to prevent cancer. My grandfather wasn't sick a day in his life and passed on from old age at the remarkable milestone age of ninety-six. Using the information in this chapter, you can incorporate supplements in your life and reap the numerous health-related rewards.

10

Psychotherapy

"The greatest discovery of my generation is that human beings can alter their lives by altering their attitudes of mind."
—WILLIAM JAMES (1842–1910)

There is a link between your emotional state and the health of your skin and hair as emotional stress can trigger stress-related conditions in both of them. Research has confirmed that therapy can help you to manage emotional distress and aid in the healing process of stress-related skin and hair conditions, especially when used in conjunction with dermatologic treatments.[1]

When you are stressed out and going through a difficult time in your life, talking to someone else can make you feel better. Sounds pretty simple, right? This is why having a best friend, family member, or significant other to confide in when times are tough is such a valuable part of the relational experience. It makes you feel better to talk to someone else, to have your feelings validated and hear their perspective on your problems. Sigmund Freud, the father of psychoanalysis, called this the *talking cure.* It was he who developed the initial tools of psychoanalysis, which used conversation to help patients uncover repressed or unconscious issues—ones he thought generally stemmed from childhood events—in order to move toward healing and change.[2] It can be incredibly helpful to talk to a therapist when you need to share your innermost issues with a person who knows how to listen in an unbiased manner, without agenda or ulterior motive, and who can offer a healthy, balanced perspective on your life. For many reasons, there are times when friends or family members, or even significant others, cannot provide the same kind of balanced perspective and guidance that a professionally trained therapist can.

In my experience, speaking with a trained professional can be extremely beneficial. Whenever I have brunch with my therapist friend Laurie, she always manages to challenge me in healthy ways. Over our meal, we exchange typical friendly banter, catch up on the kids, and then she asks me the hard questions. It is her talent for getting to the heart of a matter that makes our time together rewarding. She will ask me something deep and thought-provoking, and I will have to hold my breath and contemplate my answer. When I respond, she challenges me in ways that knock my socks off and encourages me to challenge myself. Then, as a good friend does, she refreshes my ears by telling me of her own woes. Her honesty and openness about her own problems remind me that she is not some mysterious creature able to read my mind and advise me, but another human being with flaws, issues, and difficulties, just like the individuals she treats. I value this therapeutic relationship and grow from it.

Finding a copacetic therapeutic relationship is not easy. It takes time to find the type of therapist who is the right kind of listener and advisor and who can provide a safe place for you to open up and be vulnerable. Sometimes this means you need to visit multiple therapists before discovering the right one. When you do find a beneficial therapeutic situation, you will be so glad you took the time to seek it out. Think about it: if you don't make your health and healing a priority, who will?

TYPES OF THERAPY

There are over 150 different forms of therapy. With the multitude of therapeutic techniques available today, after doing a little research, you can find the therapy that best works for you. A few popular types are described below.

Psychoanalysis

This was the beginning of Freud's *talking cure*. He believed that childhood conflicts are repressed and held in your unconscious, and this results in psychological symptoms. Talking about your past and broaching these bottled-up emotions leads to the release of harmful emotions and creates the ability to change. This technique uses free association, or saying whatever comes into your head, to look for clues that the therapist interprets.[3]

Interpersonal Psychotherapy

This *empirically proven* treatment for mood disorders theorizes that a person's depression (or other mood disorder) and life situation are related. This type of therapy seeks to uncover the disturbing life event, such as the loss of a loved one, dissolution of a relationship, loss of a job, etc., that triggered the onset of the mood disorder.[4] Or the opposite can be true—sometimes a person's mood disorder can trigger the difficult situation in their life. Once the issue is uncovered, over a short period of 12–16 weeks, this therapy seeks to help the participant resolve their feelings about the difficult life event and thereby uplift that person's mood.[5]

Cognitive Behavior Therapy (CT)

Therapists use CT to help their patients uncover irrational beliefs and negative thought processes that contribute to depression and stress, in order to help them replace harmful thoughts with positive thoughts.[6] "Research has shown that CT reduces the frequency of negative thoughts and the severity of dysfunctional attitudes, and shows that these changes are associated with depression-reduction over the course of treatment."[7] Moreover, studies have confirmed this as a beneficial form of therapy for those experiencing stress-induced skin conditions[8] and those dealing with mood disorders. CT is particularly helpful if you have anxiety or depression that causes you to pick at your skin or neglect its care, which, in turn, worsens your skin condition.

Humanistic Therapy

Humanistic therapy seeks to promote self-awareness, understanding, and acceptance in the participant. Rather than direct the course of therapy, therapists utilize empathy, unconditional warmth, and positive responses to guide participants through the process of self-actualization, which essentially means that the therapist seeks to help the participant become the best version of him or herself.[9]

Overall, the *talking cure* can help you manage your stress in a healthy way and help you to learn positive coping mechanisms. In fact, using neuroimaging techniques, researchers have found that changes occur in people's brains after they engage in psychotherapy,[10] thereby showing that therapy can promote change, both in your brain chemistry and your life. Working on yourself can lead you to heal, grow, and become the person you want to be.

PART THREE

Innovative Treatments

CHAPTERS 11–12

Chapters 11–12 describe how the innovative treatments of light-emitting diode therapy, electromagnetic field therapy, and biofeedback can promote healing. These chapters talk about the stress-induced facial conditions that will benefit from these therapies, and discuss what symptoms they treat.

11

Light-Emitting Diode Therapy

"Give light, and the darkness will disappear of itself."

—DESIDERIUS ERASMUS

Imagine you are on a space station floating in the black abyss among the stars. The majority of your time is spent moving through cramped quarters in zero gravity. How do you keep your muscles from shriveling due to lack of weight resistance? Or imagine you are stationed on a Navy submarine in the ocean depths. An accident occurs, and your arm is severely lacerated. You are miles below the surface and a continent away from a hospital. The doctor sutures you up, yet the pressure of your submerged craft slows the healing process. It was just these types of scenarios that prompted NASA to develop a technology to combat these problems. It is called light-emitting diode (LED) therapy.

Originally tried in experiments to spawn plant growth in space, LED technology showed promise for promoting healing and growth of *human* tissue by delivering light deep into tissues of the body.[1] Now, NASA uses this technology to treat "muscle and bone atrophy in astronauts."[2] NASA-sponsored studies have also used LED treatments on the wounds of crew members aboard deep-sea submarines and found they decrease healing time by 50 percent.[3] The good news is that you don't need to be an astronaut stationed in space or a sailor braving deep foreign waters to benefit from light-emitting diode treatments. Dermatologists now work with LED therapy to promote the healing of many skin maladies and diseases in regular individuals.

In the field of dermatology, LED treatments are a non-invasive light therapy. The healing powers of this technology not only promote skin rejuvenation, but also wound healing and tissue regeneration. For those severely affected by scarring,[4] rosacea, acne, psoriasis (particularly psoriasis that has not responded to other treatments), wound healing,[5] unusual rashes, hair loss,[6] sunspots, or wrinkles, LED therapy can help.[7]

When I had my palsy, I completed a session of red-light LED therapy every forty-eight hours. After each session, I felt a decrease in the ear pain I was experiencing, as well as a decrease in overall discomfort. Some days it felt like I was starting to have facial movement, even though clinically I was not. I believe this was due to the deeper muscle and nerve fibers that were starting to strengthen and react before the results could be observed because, suddenly, after three weeks of this treatment, I awoke with movement in my face. I had used several therapies during my recovery, so I may never know which of these was the most helpful, but I do believe each played a significant role in my recovery.

How Light-Emitting Diodes Work

Light-emitting diodes work through a mechanism called photobiomodulation (PBM) where cells in the body or skin absorb the light that, in turn, triggers a biochemical reaction. Once skin absorbs the light, PBM operates in several ways. It kickstarts immune functions in our cells, exerts an anti-inflammatory effect, and increases cell activities, particularly the production of collagen, a fibrous protein that connects and supports the tissue of the skin. Because it prompts skin cells to reproduce, LED therapy rejuvenates the skin and can be used to remedy wrinkles or sun-damaged cells. LED stimulates the immune system's skin-cell activity and boosts the body's natural healing process. As a result, it can reduce inflammation, clear up blemishes, kill the bacteria associated with acne, and even kill precancerous cells.

LED technology is comprised of three different types of light—red, blue, and yellow (infrared). While all types of light have positive effects and help jolt our immune system into action on the cellular level, each type has a different function.

- Red LED's decrease inflammation of the skin and penetrate deeper into the tissue. This light treatment improves the inflammation seen in psoriatic plaques. Red light is also used to treat the discoloration associated with rosacea, and treat inflammatory rashes and chemotherapy-related rashes. It can also be successfully used on sun-damaged skin, wrinkles, sunspots, and uneven colored splotches included.
- For psoriasis, a combination of LED's are used to clear the debris on the skin. A study I conducted at the Ablon Skin Institute and Research Center indicates this is a particularly beneficial treatment option if you have persistent psoriasis that does not respond to topical medication alone.[8]
- Yellow LED's penetrate deep into the skin to improve wound healing, and they help with pain, especially in the muscles or joints.
- Blue LED's are used to kill surface bacteria on the skin, and they can be used to treat acne as this light eradicates the bacteria associated with the condition. In combination with topical skin activators, such as levulanic acid, this type of light is also used to destroy precancerous lesions on the skin.

Those undergoing LED therapy will feel virtually no pain. Light-emitting diodes are very different from lasers, which work through heating the tissue. Because LED's do not heat the tissue, they cause no discomfort, swelling, or scarring. In office-treatment sessions, the light is administered through a unit that hovers over the affected area, and at home, handheld devices that cover a much smaller surface area can be used. Based on the skin condition being treated, office sessions are usually 20–30 minutes long and are conducted once or twice a week. A key benefit to this type of treatment is the fact that there is no recovery time associated with each session. After a treatment, you will be able to return to your normal schedule without having to worry about noticeable swelling or discoloration of your skin.

It is always a good idea to seek the advice of a board-certified dermatologist before beginning LED therapy to determine if this is the right course of action regarding your condition, and ensure that you are applying this therapy in the most beneficial way. For example, I rarely prescribe LED therapy alone, I almost always use it in combination with other treatments. Moreover, the duration of the therapy varies, depending on your specific skin condition.

12

Electrical Stimulation and Biofeedback

> "There are three values: Feel good, be good, and do good."
>
> –YOGI BHAJAN

Pulsed-Electromagnetic Field Therapy

Pulsed-Electromagnetic Field Therapy (PEMF) operates through short bursts of electrical current that are generated into the tissue to help wounds heal and to diminish pain and swelling. The first pulsed-radiofrequency electromagnetic field device was FDA-approved in 1950 to treat postoperative pain and swelling (edema). In the last decade, scientific data has substantiated the use of this non-invasive therapy to help with wound healing.

PEMF is an adjunctive therapy that can aid pain relief, healing, and recovery in skin conditions.[1] The short electrical bursts, that are not painful, are administered through a circular plastic covering that safely houses the wires— one side effect is that they often create a tickling sensation in the area where they are placed. Treatment sessions generally last for twenty minutes, up to three times a day, or in acute situations, they can be administered more frequently (every hour) to aid in the healing of a wound.

In my office, I have used this handheld machine for the last three years and have recommended the use of home PEMF units for my patients, who have reported that they love the reduction in pain the machine brings them. I first used this device when I had a severe sprained ankle that prevented me from exercising. I had tried other techniques to speed up my recovery, but got no results until I started using PEMF therapy. I also used this treatment for my recovery from Bell's palsy—I underwent a PEMF session every day and this helped reduce the pain in my ear and along my jawline. Research verifies that this device provides an increase in blood flow and a reduction of pain and swelling that I can also attest to.[2]

Some physicians have PEMF units in their office, but it is becoming more common for physicians to recommend that patients purchase home PEMF units, which are quite inexpensive.

Biofeedback

During biofeedback sessions, therapists attach electrical sensors (electrodes) to your skin to monitor your basic body functions—heart rate, breathing rate, blood pressure, temperature, sweating, and muscle activity—as you talk with the therapist. While you are discussing your concerns, if your heart rate increases, or your blood pressure rises, the attached electrodes will send signals to the monitor in the form of flashing lights or sounds. These signals allow your body to give you feedback when you are stressed out.[3]

The goal of biofeedback is to acknowledge what is changing in your body in response to a situation—you could be experiencing a racing heart, anger, or frustration. If your body exhibits any signs of stress during a biofeedback session, the therapist will teach you relaxation exercises and you will learn to employ the relaxation techniques to control your body functions and calm down.[4] As you calm down and your levels return to normal, the monitor allows you to see or hear the change in those vital signs.

This painless technique is a way to help you focus on converting negative emotional reactions to situations that stress or anger you into more positive, healthier reactions. It allows you to focus on breathing and relaxing, using the power of your own thoughts to control your bodily reactions.

This is one of my favorite exercises. It provides a sense of power because it allows me to harness my mind and control my own body. I first used the technique to help with the anxiety I was experiencing whenever I was faced with taking big tests like the MCAT, the admission test for medical school. Back then, my biofeedback sessions provided me with the tools to train myself to calm down, relax, and take the tests one question at a time. During medical school, I applied this relaxing technique to many things that stressed me out, including standing over cadavers that smelled of formalin in anatomy class, and taking medical school exams. And I still employ this technique now. Bringing my body to a state of calm has allowed me to succeed on many levels without having an emotional breakdown. Inexpensive, portable biofeedback gadgets can be found online to help de-stress, especially if you can't get in to see a biofeedback specialist.

It's a technique anyone can and should learn. Just think how nice it would be, while sitting in traffic, to be able to remain calm instead of getting frustrated at a situation you cannot control. A red light may just be a signal for you to reassess what is important and how useless getting yourself stressed-out can be. Your body is speaking to you when you experience a racing heart or stress, and it is important to learn to listen to it and practice calming down.

PART FOUR

Non-Invasive Skin Treatments and Procedures

CHAPTERS 13–14

Chapter 13 describes the over-the-counter skin and hair products and prescription medications that are beneficial for treating stress-induced facial conditions, and provides recommendations for what types of creams and ointments to use to treat wrinkles, rejuvenate skin, and stimulate hair growth. Chapter 14 unpacks how non-invasive skin and hair procedures work to treat stress-induced conditions.

13

Over-the-Counter Products and Prescription Medications

"We must take situations as they are. We must only change our mental attitudes towards them."

–MAHARISHI MAHESH YOGI

The question I am asked on a daily basis is, "Do over-the-counter skin creams and hair products really do anything?" Well, just as prescription skin and hair products *do* something, so do many topical over-the-counter skin and hair topical products, such as creams, lotions, ointments, gels, foams, and shampoos. These products are referred to as cosmeceuticals—a term coined by the brilliant dermatologist and chemist, Dr. Albert Kingman, more than thirty years ago—because they utilize a combination of cosmetic and pharmaceutical technology and claim to have medical benefits. In this chapter, I will discuss what ingredients to look for in your cosmeceutical skin and hair products and provide an overview of prescription medications that are beneficial for stress-induced skin and hair conditions.

The effectiveness of cosmeceutical skin and hair products generally depends on a formula with three key components.

- The size of the molecule that makes up the product is important. For example, in moisturizers the molecules need to be small enough to penetrate the skin. If the molecules that comprise the moisturizer are too large, they will just sit on the surface of the skin and have superficial effects. The same concept applies to hair products, as the molecules in the formula need to be small enough to sink into the skin and then become incorporated into the hair follicles.
- A successful formula also needs a sufficiently high concentration of active ingredients in the product to actually change the composition of your skin or hair.
- Lastly, the type of substance used as the vehicle to carry the active ingredient into the skin/hair follicle is crucial to a formula's success because it helps determine whether the product can penetrate the skin's barrier. In the following section, I will break down the ingredients in skin and hair products and use them as a guide to choosing effective cosmeceutical products.

Cosmeceutical Skincare Products

With the advance of technology, the ability to make skin products that penetrate deep into the skin's barrier increases. Currently, my research center, the Ablon Skin Institute, is conducting studies to develop a technology that will enhance the absorption of skincare products into the skin. This will allow the products to reach down to lower tissue levels and stimulate new cell production, DNA repair, and collagen remodeling, thereby creating younger, rejuvenated skin.

The following section will describe skin products that have been scientifically proven to work and new skin products currently under development. Not every type of product is right for all skin types, so it's a good idea to discuss your potential choices with your dermatologist before choosing one.

Sunscreens

The most important anti-aging tool available is sunscreen. I tell my patients, if you only use one thing, sunscreen should be it. Put it by your toothpaste, so you remember to use it every morning. Even when it's cloudy outside, harmful ultraviolet light is still coming through. When shopping for a sunscreen product, look for a sun protection factor (SPF) of at least 30 that blocks out ultraviolet A (UVA) light. Also look for the ingredients of zinc oxide or avobenzone—Parsol 1789—that block the majority of ultraviolet B light. Zinc is a physical block, and this means it provides instant coverage once applied. Avobenzone is a chemical block, which means it takes about 20 minutes to activate and provide coverage. Each individual has their own threshold at which they tan and then burn, so if your skin is burning using a SPF of 30 or below, you should use a sunscreen with a higher SPF. While many people are aware that burning is a sign of sun damage, most are not aware that tanning is also a sign of sun damage. So slather up with sunscreen (and take oral vitamin D, so you won't be deficient in it from lack of sun exposure).

Moisturizers

Keep it simple and try to find a sunscreen/moisturizer rolled into one, so you can save a step in your skincare regimen. Moisturizers are important for those who are dealing with eczema or dry skin. Whenever you try a new moisturizer, or any skin product, you want to test a little behind your ear and wait a while to make sure you are not allergic (generally one to three days).

The types of ingredients to look for when picking a moisturizer are outlined below. Look for moisturizes that have ingredients from each category.

- **Occlusive ingredients.** These create a film on the surface of skin to block water loss (i.e. petrolatum, paraffin, dimethicone, or silicone derivatives, cetyl alcohol, stearyl alcohol, stearic acid, lanolin, or propylene glycol).

- **Humectant ingredients.** These attract water from the inside of your skin and trap water from the environment (i.e. glycerin, honey, ammonium lactate, urea, propylene glycol, hyaluronic acid, sorbitol, panthenol, sodium pyrrolidine, carboxylic acid, or sodium PCA).
- **Emollient ingredients.** These provide a smooth texture to the skin as they act like caulking to fill the cracks between the cells and wrinkles (i.e. isopropyl isostearate, propylene glycol, octyl stearate, jojoba oil, dimethicone, octyl octanoate, isopropyl palmitate, or isostearyl alcohol).
- **Retinoids** (retinol, retinaldehyde, retinyl esters, and retinoic acid). Retinoids and vitamin-A derivatives are generally found in antiaging products. These ingredients help many skin conditions, including sun-damaged skin caused by long-term exposure to sunlight (sunspots) and aging skin (wrinkles), psoriasis, acne, actinic keratosis (skin growths that often turn into cancer), and many other skin conditions. They work by thickening the layer of skin known as the epidermis, turning over dead cells, and stimulating collagen production. There are many retinoid skin products that are available over the counter. Only retinoic acid is by prescription.[1]
- **Vitamin C.** This is a naturally occurring antioxidant, generally found in cream or ointment form, that is used to prevent and treat sun damage to the skin, including sunspots and wrinkles. Ultraviolet light alters DNA, cell membranes, collagen, and other proteins in the skin, which results in sun-damaged skin and causes oxidative stress. Vitamin C, an antioxidant, not only protects the skin from the harmful effects of ultraviolet light, but also has anti-inflammatory effects, and helps with the synthesis of collagen. Taking this vitamin orally can help the skin, but it is more effective to apply it topically to the skin. Newer versions of vitamin-C ointments and creams are less irritating and use refined technology, which leads to greater skin improvement and fewer side effects. Look for a

serum that has L-ascorbic acid (the most active form of vitamin C) and a minimum concentration of 10 percent.

- **Vitamin B.** Specifically, vitamins B_3 (niacinamide) and B_5 (panthenol) that can be found in anti-aging, acne, and moisturizing skin products. These vitamins have been shown to help aging (texture and wrinkles) and sun-damaged skin (sunspots), as well as acne. They also help with wound healing and act as a moisturizer and antioxidant. Vitamin B_3 has also been shown to improve the skin's ability to act as a barrier, decrease facial erythema (redness), hyperpigmentation (brown and black spots), and yellowing skin.[2]
- **Botanicals** (plant extracts). American Indians first demonstrated the medicinal properties of plant extracts to the European settlers hundreds of years ago. Although plant extracts may be all-natural, they must undergo substantial chemical processing prior to being incorporated into skincare products, and this may influence their potential effectiveness. Botanical extracts can be found in cleansers, moisturizers, and anti-aging creams, and can help with aging, inflammation, and even skin cancer.

Below is a list of botanical extracts to look for in your skin products.

BENEFITS OF BOTANICAL EXTRACTS

Botanical antioxidants. Soy, curcumin, silymarin, pycnogenol. resveratrol.[3]

Botanical anti-inflammatories. Ginkgo biloba, green tea, witch-hazel, tea tree, lavender, chamomile, grapeseed, arnica, echinacea, white willow, lavender, saw palmetto, borage, green tea, evening primrose.

Botanical skin-soothing agents. Prickly pear, aloe vera, allantoin, witch-hazel, papaya, oat straw, flax, fenugreek, slippery elm, resveratrol (also called the "Longevity Molecule").[4]

Botanical anti-aging. Soy, grapeseed, pomegranate, green and black tea, avocado, garlic, resveratrol.[5]

Botanical anti-skin-cancer. Rosemary, ginseng, silymarin, green/black/white tea, garlic, ginger, and pomegranate.

New botanical algae products. Algae extracts from seaweed contain an ingredient known as alguronic acid that has shown promise as an antioxidant, anti-inflammatory, and exfoliant to smooth, moisturize, and rejuvenate skin.[6]

Metals

Metals have been used in skincare for over 3,500 years. The most common metals found in skincare products are listed here.

- **Zinc.** Found in sunscreens and topical soothing agents, including skin products for babies. Zinc is often used in baby products to soothe baby's bottoms. Scientific data shows that zinc has wound-healing properties and acts as an anti-inflammatory and antioxidant.
- **Copper.** Found in many skin moisturizers and anti-aging products. A copper-rich diet can reduce oxidative stress, act as an antioxidant, and help heal wounds. Skincare products have subsequently incorporated this metal to potentially have the same effect on the skin. The only issue is that copper molecules are quite large, making absorption into the skin difficult.[7]
- **Selenium.** This metal is found in acne, antioxidant skin creams, and anti-aging skin products because of its ability to reduce collagen damage from the sun and act as an antioxidant. Selenium can also reduce the risk of non-melanoma skin cancers when taken orally and can reduce the risk of skin tumors when applied topically.[8]

Peptides

These are small proteins that can help reduce wrinkles and firm the skin without causing irritation. Peptides are found in anti-aging products, and products based on this technology are generally less expensive than other anti-aging products. Scientists are now able to make small fragments of peptides that can stimulate the production of collagen and elastin (the structural base of skin). There are several types of peptides. While some work to stimulate the enzymes needed in collagen production, others mimic neuromodulators (botulinum toxin like Botox, Dysport, Myobloc, or Xeomin) and soften dynamic wrinkles, or those caused from repeated muscle movement (smile lines). In your anti-aging products, look for hexapeptides (6 ring peptides) that work on dynamic wrinkles, and pentapeptides (5 ring peptides) that work on collagen production.[9]

Hydroxyl Acid Exfoliants

Hydroxyl acids can be used for treating acne, dry skin, scarring, precancerous lesions, and sun damage. This type of product dates back to 45 B.C. In fact, Cleopatra bathed in sour milk (which contained lactic acid) to exfoliate her skin and make it look radiant and beautiful. Frequently, hydroxyl acids are used in conjunction with lightening agents to even out irregularities in skin pigmentation. There are two types of hydroxyl acids—alpha and beta—and of the two, beta hydroxy acid is the least irritating.[10]

Skin-Lightening Agents

Hyperpigmentation, or dark spots on the skin, can result from hormonal changes, acne, shingles, and sun damage. Topical treatments for dark spots are recently stepping into the forefront of research. Skin-lightening products range from prescription strength to over-the-counter natural lightening ingredients. A few are discussed on the following pages.

- **Hydroquinone.** This phenol-based compound has received a lot of negative press, but it remains the most successful topical lightener available today. Lower concentrations have been available over the counter but when the prescription-strength varieties (ranging from 4–10 percent) are combined with retinoic acid or hydroxyl acid, they cannot be beat for improving all forms of hyperpigmentation (especially melasma). Rare complications occur with this topical, so I recommend taking a break from it after a few months use.
- **Kojic acid.** Derived from fungal elements, this lightening agent (used to prevent the browning of food items) works best when combined with hydroxyl acids and corticosteroids, as it can be quite irritating.
- **Licorice extract.** The active ingredient here is glabridin, and this product also works best in combination with such acids as kojic acid, vitamin C, and arbutin.
- **Soy.** This evens skin discoloration by a different mechanism than the products mentioned above, but it is only present in fresh soy, not pasteurized soy milk.
- **Arbutin.** This extract from bearberry fruits has mild skin-lightening properties and is added to many lightening products.
- **Vitamin C.** This is not only an antioxidant but it also lightens skin by stopping pigment production in melanin synthesis.
- **Hydroxy acids.** They speed up cell turnover to increase and improve all skin lighteners by increasing product absorption.[8,9]

Endogenous Growth Factors

Anti-aging creams now use this technology, which was initially studied for use in wound healing. Since sun-damaged skin is similar to a wound, this technology can be used to repair sun-damaged skin as it mimics the qualities of young skin and renews aging skin.[11,12,13]

Enzyme Technology

Used in extracts, creams, and masks to repair damaged skin. When you are young, your body has the enzymes to repair damage to the skin. As people age, these enzymes decrease and the skin's ability to repair itself fails. Topical enzyme therapy replaces these much needed enzymes to boost skin repair and protection levels in order to defend against aging skin and DNA damage.

Stem-Cell Technology

This anti-aging product is typically derived from stem-cell extracts from non-embryonic human cells, similar to extracting a person's own stem cells from fat that has been removed (liposuction), and then re-injecting it. There are also new products coming to the market from other sources, including embryonic and umbilical-cord stem cells. This type of product is generally found as a stem-cell serum, ointment, or cream. It accelerates the creation of skin cells, which results in smoother, younger, healthier skin. Stem cells are also being investigated for their use in hair-growth stimulation. New research studies out of Japan are demonstrating an even easier way to generate stem cells through exposure to acidic environments in the lab. This means more access to stem cells, which can be used to not only improve your skin, but also regenerate organs and even reverse genetic aging.[14] There is more: a new company, NuGene Inc, in Costa Mesa, California that is now able to take a person's harvested fat cells (removed through a local anesthetic without pain), and create a personalized nanotechnology serum or cream using stem-cell technology.

Glycobiology

This new technology incorporates sugar chains or glycans into skin cosmeceuticals, such as anti-aging serums and moisturizers. Glycans, or sugars in skin tissue, decrease with aging, as a result, moisturizers containing these sugars are being developed. The first one was launched in 2012.[15]

Proteases

These enzymes are currently found in cleansers and moisturizers. They reduce pro-inflammatory proteins, improve the skin's ability to repair its outer layer, and decrease scaling, itching, and redness. This is great for the stress-induced skin conditions of psoriasis, eczema, and rosacea, but be aware that allergic reactions can be a risk.[16]

Telomeres

This anti-aging technology is currently being developed. Telomeres are the genetic material within your cells that act as the cell's ticking clock. As telomeres shorten, the cell dies. It has been shown that stressed women have shorter telomeres, meaning their cells age faster.[17] Current studies are investigating how telomere technology can reduce DNA damage and cell aging without promoting abnormal cells growth.[18,19,20]

Prescription Drugs

Prescription drugs for stress-induced skin conditions are listed here.

- **Azelaic acid.** This topical prescription, a lightening and anti-acne product derived from a yeast, works well on rosacea, as well as on dark spots left by old acne. The main side effect seems to be dryness.
- **Barrier-repair medication.** Barrier deficiencies in the skin are one of the underlying causes of eczema/atopic dermatitis. Those with eczema have leaky skin cells, which increase water loss and the ability of toxins to permeate the skin. This type of medication can repair the barrier of the skin and protect against these issues,[21] as well as help to reduce itching and secondary infection from scratching.
- **Corticosteroids** (steroids). This medication can be applied topically to the skin, taken orally, or injected. It works to calm the

skin in those who are experiencing inflammation due to eczema, psoriasis, rosacea, or Bell's palsy. It also reduces the itching associated with these disorders. It should be noted that long-term use of these steroids could actually slow the skin's ability to repair its barrier because it thins the skin and causes broken capillaries, subsequently leading to flare-ups of the condition being treated.[22]

- **Dovonex.** Topical vitamin D ointment for psoriasis, which is believed to regulate the immune system.[23] Vitamin D deficiency is frequently seen in people who have psoriasis or many other autoimmune diseases, but the use of a vitamin D ointment or cream may not be enough to reverse the deficiency of this vitamin. No significant side effects, but not always a successful form of treatment.
- **Metronidazole.** This topical antibiotic and anti-parasitic agent is used for the treatment of rosacea and results in some improvement for some individuals. It is believed to reduce the inflammation associated with rosacea. I typically will not use this medication as the sole therapy to treat rosacea.
- **Retinoic acid** or tazarotene (the strongest of all the retinoids). Great for the treatment of acne, psoriasis, plaques, sun damage, and wrinkles. The main side effect is dryness and irritation, so it should be applied sparingly, every other day, or even every third day.

Cosmeceutical Hair Products

There have been many innovations in hair products that help with hair loss or thinning hair. The most effective types are described below and range from holistic to over-the-counter cosmeceuticals, to prescription products.

Holistic Preparations

- **Botanicals for hair loss** (alopecia). Thyme, rosemary, cedarwood, grapeseed, jojoba, apple, Dabao or Chinese herbs, saw palmetto.
- **Metals**

  Copper sprays are a great addition to a hair-care regimen especially in cases of hair thinning or hair loss. The copper works here to reduce inflammation, which allows hair to grow.

  Selenium in hair-care products can help to reduce inflammation of the hair follicles, which can allow hair to grow.

Over-the-Counter Preparations

- **Minoxidil** (Rogaine). Topical minoxidil is now an over-the-counter product that comes in concentrations of 2 percent and 5 percent. The lower concentration is made for women, specifically of child-bearing age. Even though I frequently recommend the higher concentration for better results, I also caution that, for women, the higher-concentration formula can cause hair growth in undesired male hair-bearing areas. If this topical does work for you, it's a lifelong commitment. Any hair growth seen with minoxidil will fall out if you cease use of the product. While the medicine appears to prolong the hair-growth phase, other mechanisms of action are possible, including increased blood supply to the scalp, but as of yet, how this product works is still undetermined. In my office, women do seem to respond better to the product than men. In my clinical experience, it tends to prevent women from losing more hair, as opposed to creating new hair growth. The side effects are few and uncommon, and my patients tolerate the topical well, even if the application tip may be a little annoying and cumbersome. Be aware that this product takes approximately three to six months to see results, and must be continued on an indefinite basis if it does work. Minoxidil is not to be used on women who are pregnant or breastfeeding, as there are no studies showing it is safe for these groups to use.

- **Viviscal.** This is an all-natural protein extract from deep-sea fish that is enriched with vitamins. It works to slow hair loss, increase terminal hair growth, and increase hair diameter for fuller, thicker hair. These results are verified by a just-completed study at the Ablon Skin Institute and Research Center on hair-diameter changes in patients taking Viviscal.[24] Supplements are taken twice a day for approximately six months, even though the center has seen increased hair growth in just three months in its studies.[25] Once people are happy with the amount of hair they have grown, they can reduce their pill intake to once a day, sometimes even less frequently. Studies have yet to be conducted to determine the optimal frequency that the medication should be taken.
- **Topical Biomimetic Peptide HRS-10** (acetyl tetrapeptide-3). This peptide is mixed with red clover extract, which is rich in Biochanin and helps prevent hair loss, slow hair thinning, and stimulate new hair growth. It also reduces damage caused by inflammation, providing fuller, thicker, and healthier looking hair.

Prescriptions

- **Corticosteroids** (steroids). Multiple injections are placed directly into the areas of hair loss, reducing inflammation at the site of hair follicles, and allowing hair to grow.
- **Oral finasteride.** This medication has more side effects than the steroid injections, but is one of the more effective agents for hair growth. It works by decreasing the production of DHT, leading to slower hair loss and increased hair growth. It generally takes at least three months to see any results. This medication is not safe for women of childbearing age. Side effects include sexual dysfunction, dizziness, and rashes, as well as changes in the level of

prostate hormones in men. I have a pharmacy create a topical finasteride mixture for my patients that has fewer side effects, but the lower dosage may also lower the effectiveness.

- **Spironolactone.** Not only does this medication help acne, but because it lowers androgen production, it also can help hair (both excess and loss). It is a relatively safe medication but since it is a diuretic, it is important to avoid potassium-rich foods, such as bananas, and watch for irregular menses in women. While it is not first line in my treatment of hair loss or hirsutism, it is a useful treatment method.

New Technology

My lab, the Ablon Skin Institute and Research Center, is currently testing a new topical growth stimulator for hair. Also on the horizon are treatments, such as topical 5-alfa-reductase inhibitors, that prevent the body from converting the male sex hormone testosterone into the type of hormone that triggers hair loss. Platelet-rich protein has recently been used to stimulate hair growth, but scientific proof is still not available.

As technology continues to improve at a rapid pace, so does the effectiveness of skin and hair products. Oftentimes, finding the product that works for you begins with understanding the types of creams, serums, ointments, and prescriptions available on the market today. There are so many products on the shelf, it can be overwhelming to choose one that will actually make a difference for you, but fortified by the knowledge provided in this chapter, you have help making purchasing decisions that count, so you will start seeing a difference in your skin and hair.

14

Non-Invasive Procedures

"As human beings, our greatness lies not so much in being able to remake the world—that is the myth of the atomic age—as in being able to remake ourselves."

—MAHATMA GANDHI

It seems that everyone is curious about non-invasive procedures and the newest technologies available. At my lectures, or in my office, this is always a topic of interest. The technology for non-invasive procedures is advancing rapidly, opening up a wide array of options that offer dramatic results. Many people benefit from these types of procedures. Years of sun exposure, stress-induced skin-disorders, and menopause all thin the top layer of your skin and generally lead to a breakdown in the structural proteins, collagen, and elastin in the deeper layer of your skin, as well as causing sunspots and broken capillaries. Non-invasive procedures can repair damaged skin and turn back the clock, making you look years younger, all with minimal-to-no recovery time. Below are descriptions of the newest and most effective procedures.

Photorejuvenation

Almost every individual at some age will have some degree of sun damage. Even if you wear sunscreen, you will still absorb some sunlight (often not enough is applied, or not reapplied, or it's not sunny, so you don't put any sunscreen on). Photorejuvenation, performed with an intense pulsed light (IPL), is not a true laser, and has filters that allow certain wavelengths to pass through, while blocking out others. Treatments are modified based on skin type, as well as the kind of damage treated (sunspots, broken capillaries, collagen tightening, and acne, or rosacea). This treatment can dramatically improve the flushing (from broken capillaries) associated with the skin conditions such as rosacea and eczema. When people experience a clearing in their skin, they often feel emotionally uplifted as a result. A new study out of Stanford showed that women who completed around six sessions throughout the year, looked as young as they had five-to-eleven years earlier when they began the study.[1]

This is a relatively simple procedure that requires four-to-six sessions performed once a month, after which, a single treatment for maintenance every six months will be needed. There is an exciting benefit from this procedure as it also destroys some excess facial hair. For this reason, if you have ingrown hairs, this is a great treatment. Men who want to grow a full beard may want to avoid the beard area in sessions.

There is little recovery time needed after a photorejuvenation session; however, I do tell my patients that, depending on the amount of damage, after the first few sessions their skin may look like a chocolate chip cookie, but this can usually be covered with makeup. This treatment can literally make you look and feel ten years younger, and can be performed on almost every part of the body. I get photorejuvenation once a year for maintenance.

Radiofrequency

Radiofrequency devices use heat on body areas, such as love handles, tummy, and buttocks, or on the face to dissolve fat and tighten skin. The types of devices include monopolar, bipolar, and even tripolar. In my opinion, the monopolar and bipolar devices can be uncomfortable, and sometimes the temperature can even be intolerable. The newer versions of radiofrequency units allow for delivery of heat to a focused area and let the administrator observe the desired temperature of the skin during the procedure, so it never gets too hot, or too uncomfortable, yet is still effective in tightening the skin and dissolving fat.

This procedure is generally performed every two weeks for 6–8 sessions. There is absolutely no downtime or recovery time needed with any of the radiofrequency devices. Depending on the results you desire, maintenance sessions will be needed once every 2–6 months. I am a fan of this device because, after two kids, no amount of sit-ups seems to tighten that skin around the belly, but this procedure will.

Infrared Lasers and Light Sources

These devices are specifically designed to tighten skin. Both the infrared lasers and infrared light sources bypass the surface of the skin and go directly into the deeper tissue layer to treat the collagen and elastin fibers of the dermis. Heating these fibers tightens the skin and initiates new collagen formation, but because the surface of the skin is left untouched, there is no downtime or recovery time needed. Typically only two sessions are needed two months apart. Once a year, or every two years, a maintenance session is suggested. This procedure works very well for aging skin, skin laxity (bags, jowls), and wound healing (for which it is performed 2–3 times a week until healing is complete). I find when the skin under my eyes looks tired and wrinkled, one quick session with this virtually painless machine tightens things right up, and the results last about a year-and-a-half.

Fillers

As you age and are exposed to the sun, you begin to lose fullness in the face, neck décolleté, and hands. Have you ever marveled at how cherubic a baby's face looks, and wondered why you lost this youthful essence in your own face as you aged? Over time, the fat and fullness of the face deteriorates, leading to a loss of that cherubic essence. Fillers can immediately replenish that missing fullness, and can actually rejuvenate the skin by stimulating permanent collagen production. When you return the following year for more fillers, you may find that, even though the filler has diminished, your lines are not as deep as they were before. New types of fillers lead to this result as they stimulate the production of permanent collagen as they dissolve and, as the filler is placed, the needle pricks also stimulate collagen production, called collagen-induction therapy (CIT).

There are permanent, semi-permanent, and temporary fillers available, including types that can be dissolved if you dislike the look. New fillers are lasting up to two years and the collagen-induction therapy allows for a permanent or long-lasting effect. When fillers are placed correctly, there are no lumps or bumps, and it results in smooth, younger looking skin. However, bruising can occur. In my office, I hand out a *Before and After Tip Sheet* to reduce the risk of bruising. These tips include eating pineapple, or bromelin, an enzyme that occurs naturally in pineapples, before injections, and avoiding aspirin or ibuprofen afterwards.

While recovery time is not needed after these procedures, you may have some bruising, so don't get this done right before a big party or photo shoot. The results you get from fillers really do depend on the doctor administering the procedure. When done correctly, this procedure can turn back the clock and make you look as you did 10–20 years ago. It takes a truly artistic hand to create a fantastic look that is not overfilled or overdone. For this reason, when you go to a dermatologist or cosmetic surgeon, check to see if the staff gets fillers performed by their doctor, and make sure you like the way they look and the way the doctor looks. You don't want your lips to enter a room before you do, so my philosophy is always to start conservatively and then add more if needed. A recent study demonstrated that those who had their fillers topped off 6–9 months after the initial procedure, had results that lasted 18–21 months.[2]

Neuromodulators—Vitamin B or D

Neuromodulators, which are botulinum toxins, have literally transformed people's lives. A large study found that those with moderate to severe wrinkles experienced an overall improvement in their quality of life after receiving treatments.[3] Not only do they treat dynamic wrinkles (lines that appear with facial movement: smile lines, frown lines), they also treat migraines, excess sweating, and many neurologic disorders. I found neuromodulators extremely helpful in improving the symmetry of my face during my palsy, especially pertaining to evening out the height of my eyebrows. If you have any permanent nerve damage, you can find dramatic improvement in the symmetry of your face. When you look in the mirror, the defect will be less noticeable, and people will stare less. Emotionally, your confidence can be lifted and the results can be maintained with near-painless injections every 4–6 months. In general, this treatment can erase 5–10 years off your face.

My patients always ask if I do this procedure on myself. I find that over the years I do it less and less because my goal is not to freeze my face, or anyone else's for that matter, but rather to soften those lines that appear due to recurring facial movement. When I utilize neuromodulators, I look less angry with my kids, and less wrinkled when I glance in the mirror, but I can certainly still smile, frown, and look surprised. My favorite place for these injections is actually around my lips. I have naturally full lips, but lip lines appear no matter how hard you try to prevent them. A little amount of filler goes a long way, and while I can't play the flute (fillers can interfere with this), those lip lines never looked better. And when I tell my patients what I've done, they are surprised and can't believe how natural my vitamin-D neuromodulator looks. It's not for everyone though, especially musicians. Targeted cold therapy, as well as botulinum toxin creams/serums are now being developed as treatments to soften lines and wrinkles, in conjunction with some neuromodulator injections or for those who are needle-phobic.

Laser Hair Removal

There have been remarkable advances in hair removal for all skin types and hair colors. Laser wavelengths are extremely pigmentation specific. Now, due to innovations in technology, people of all ethnicities who have excess hair growth can be treated, just as the longer wavelengths can be used to treat darker skin types. Hair-removal lasers now also work on all types of hair colors. If hair is red, blonde, or gray, a new topical solution can be applied to the root of the hair allowing it to hold pigment, so it will respond to the laser treatment. In order for hair removal to be permanent, it is important to address the underlying cause of excess hair growth. Lasers are also a great option for any unwanted hair growth that occurs with age. This is something I'm sure my grandmother would have liked (I used to pluck her chin hairs for her). I have also found this procedure helpful as I used to shave twice a day (I got that from my dad), but now that I've completed three sessions of hair removal, I haven't had to shave in sixteen years. I will certainly offer laser hair removal to my kids when they are older. There is little-to-no recovery time with this procedure, but sometimes crusting can occur at the sites of dead hair follicles, or redness or swelling that usually lasts only a few days to a week.[4]

Low Level (Light) Laser Therapy (LLLT)

This type of therapy delivers low levels of red and near-infrared light, which are lower in energy density than is seen in routine laser therapy. LLLT has also been called the *cold laser* because the density is low enough that it does not heat the tissue. This treatment can be used to do a number of things, including stimulate hair growth, heal wounds, and reduce pain, inflammation, swelling, and fat cells. LLLT is also used to treat neurologic disorders. In addition to the aforementioned uses, we utilize LLLT in my office to treat the pain associated with shingles, among a number of other things. Treatments vary from 15–40 minutes in length. For fat reduction, wound healing, and reduced pain, sessions are needed 1–2 times a week for six weeks, and sessions lasting up to six months are needed to stimulate hair growth.[5] There is no recovery time associated with this procedure.

Microneedling

Needle abrasion was developed in the early 1990s, but the first marketed microneedle system used for collagen stimulation and acne scars came about in 2004. Now this treatment is used to treat scarring (acne or in general), rejuvenate skin, and reduce wrinkles. Only in the past few years has it been possible to harness the use of this small tool to deliver truly amazing active ingredients, such as stem cells, into the skin to enhance this treatment's ability to rejuvenate the skin. When used to carry stem-cell cytokine technology into the skin, the micropunctures allow the stem-cell products to get into the deeper skin level of the dermis and stimulate the formation of new cells and new collagen and elastin. These skin punctures also cause collagen-induction therapy. You can receive these treatments every 3–4 weeks with very little downtime and few side effects, possibly a few pinpoint scabs at worst.[6]

Microneedling is a relatively new skincare procedure. It can make your skin look smoother and fresher, as well as help improve its pigmentation and texture. Studies that combine microneedling with stem-cell skincare products are currently underway at the Ablon Skin Institute and Research Center and hopefully someday this procedure can be used to change your genetic profile—making your genes younger.

Concluding Thought

As Yogi Maharishi Mahesh says:

> *"Love opens all doors, no matter how closed they may be, no matter how rusty from lack of use. Your work is to bring unity and harmony, to open all doors which have been closed for a long time. Have patience and tolerance. Open your heart all the time."*

So live, love, and find a way to reduce your stress and find a life you, your face, your skin, and your body will truly enjoy living.

Resources

Organizations

American Academy of Dermatology
Website: aad.org
Ph: 866-503-SKIN (7546)
International: 847-240-1280

National Alopecia Areata Foundation
Website: naaf.org
Ph: 415-472-3780

American Hair Loss Association
Website: americanhairloss.org
23679 Calabasas Road # 682
Calabasas, CA 91301-1502

National Eczema Association
Website: nationaleczema.org
Ph: 800-818-7546;
415-499-3474

National Institute of Neurological Disorders and Stroke
Website: ninds.nih.gov
Ph: 800-352-9424; 301-496-5751

National Psoriasis Foundation
Website: psoriasis.org
Ph: 800-723-9166

National Rosacea Society
Website: rosacea.org
Ph: 888-NO-BLUSH (662-5874)

Products

Ivivi Pulsed Electromagnetic Field Home Units: Sofpulse and Sofpulse Duo
Website: www.sofpulse.com
Ph: 415-814-2460

PEMF devices aid in healing many stress-induced facial conditions and help with pain management. Can be purchased by prescription or from a doctor's office.

Puritan's Pride
Website: Puritan.com
Ph: 800-645-3100

They have a large variety of supplements listed on their website and in their catalog.

Viviscal Supplement
Website: www.viviscal.com
Ph: 888-444-9073

An excellent supplement that supports hair growth for those experiencing hair loss or thinning hair. Can be found at CVS and Walgreens. We sell Professional Strength in our office and it can be obtained there or through other distributors.

Kim Fowler's DVDs (Founder YAS)
Website: http://go2yas.com
Ph: 866-YAS-YOGA (927-9642)

Yoga for Athletes, Yoga and Weights: A workout that explores breath and movement techniques, which are helpful in managing stress.

Perimenopausal AM/PM and Menopausal AM/PM

This supplement provides nutrients that support the hormonal changes occurring prior to and during menopause. In addition to the nationwide company listed below, these supplements are available at assorted nutrition/health stores, or in doctor's offices. We sell it in our office and you can get it online.

Whole Foods
Website: wholefoodsmarket.com
Ph: 855-265-1070

Free Smart Phone Apps

These apps provide beginners with meditation and relaxation techniques to aid in stress-management.

Darrin Marks Harmony App

Relax Melodies

Headspace

Stress check

Cleveland Clinic Stress Meditations

iSleep Easy

Yogic Breath

Endnotes

Introduction

1. Goldberg, J. "The Effects of Stress on Your Body." WebMD. Last modified July 23, 2012. Accessed June 18, 2013.

2. Ibid.

3. Ibid.

4. Woolston, C. "Of Course You are Stressed. Just Look at You." *Los Angeles Times,* April 27, 2013.

5. Ibid.

6. National Rosacea Society. "Rosacea Triggers Survey." Rosacea.org. Accessed April 22, 2013.

7. National Psoriasis Foundation. "About Psoriasis Statistics." Last modified 2013. Accessed April 22, 2013.

8. Heller, MM, Lee, ES, et al. "Stress as an Influencing Factor in Psoriasis." Skin Therapy Letter. SkinTherapyLetter.com. Last modified 06 21, 2012. Accessed June 17, 2013.

Chapter 1. Stress and Skin

1. "Stress and Skin." American Academy of Dermatology. http://www.aad.org. Last modified 2013. Accessed April 22, 2013.

2. National Psoriasis Foundation. "About Psoriasis Statistics." Last modified 2013. Accessed April 22, 2013.

3. Heller, MM, et al. "Stress as an Influencing Factor in Psoriasis." Skin Therapy Letter. SkinTherapyLetter.com. Last modified 06 21, 2012. Accessed June 17, 2013.

4. Ibid.

5. Stewart, SL. "Breaking the Psoriasis –Stress Connection." National Psoriasis Foundation. *Psoriasis Advance.* 35–39, Summer 2014.

6. Ablon, G. "Combination 830-nm and 633-nm Light-Emitting Diode Phototherapy Shows Promise in the Treatment of Recalcitrant Psoriasis: Preliminary Findings." *Photomedicine and Laser Surgery.* 28(2):141–146, 2010.

7. Millsop, JW, Bhavnit, K, Bhatia, BA, et al. "Diet and Psoriasis, Part III: Role of Nutritional Supplements." *Journal of the American Academy of Dermatology.* 561–569, September 2014.

5. Ibid.

6. Ablon, G. "Combination 830-nm and 633-nm Light-Emitting Diode Phototherapy Shows Promise in the Treatment of Recalcitrant Psoriasis: Preliminary Findings." *Photomedicine and Laser Surgery.* 28(2):141–146, 2010.

7. Wilkin, J, Dahl, M, Detmar, M, et al. "Standard grading system for rosacea: Report of the National Rosacea Society Expert Committee on the Classification and Staging of Rosacea" *Journal of the American Academy of Dermatology.* 50(6): http://www.rosacea.org/grading/gradingsystem.php. 2004.

8. Ibid.

9. Drake, L. "H. pylori Might or Might Not Trigger Rosacea." *National Rosacea Society Newsletter.* Rosacea.org. Accessed October 9, 2013.

10. Forton, FM, "Papulopustular Rosacea, Skin Immunity and Demodex: Pityriasis Folliculorum as a Missing Link." *Journal of the European Academy of Dermatology and Venereology.* 26(1):19–28, 2012.

doi: 10.1111/j.1468–3083,.2011.04310.x.

11. "Rosacea Triggers Survey." National Rosacea Society. Rosacea.org. Accessed April 22, 2013.

12. Xu, ZR, Hu, CH, Xia, MS, et al. "Effects of dietary fructooligosaccharide on digestive enzyme activities, intestinal microflora and morphology of male broilers." *Poultry Science.* 82(6):1030–1036, June 2003.

13. Otsuka, A. Doi, H, Egawa, G., et al. "Possible new therapeutic strategy to regulate atopic dermatitis through upregulating filaggrin expression." *Journal Allergy and Clinical Immunology.* pii: S0091–6749(13): 01152–01154, 2013.

14. Thuerk, S. "Researchers ID underlying cause of atopic dermatitis." *Dermatology Times.* February 27, 2014. http://dermatologytimes.modernmedicine.com/dermatology-times/news/researchers-id-underlying-cause-atopic-dermatitis

15. Buske-Kirschbaum, A, Hellhammer, DH. "Endocrine and Immune Responses to Stress in Chronic Inflammatory Skin Disorders." *Annals of the New York Academy of Sciences.* 993:231–240, 2003.

16. Hon, KL, Leung, AK, Barankin, B. "Barrier Repair Therapy in Atopic Dermatitis: An

Overview." *American Journal of Clinical Dermatology.* 14(5) doi: 10.1007/s40257-013-0033-9. 389–399, 2013.

17. Foolad, N, Brezinski, EA, Chase, EP, et al. "Effect of Nutrient Supplementation on Atopic Dermatitis in Children A Systematic Review of Probiotics, Prebiotics, Formula, and Fatty Acids." *Journal of the American Medical Association (JAMA) Dermatology.* 149(3):350–355, 2013. doi: 10.1001/jamadermatol.2013.1495 (accessed October 25, 2013).

18. "Shingles vaccination pros and cons: Vaccination against the chickenpox virus prevents a painful rash common in older men, but it has limits." *Harvard Men's Health Watch.* (11):4. June 18, 2014.

19. Park, KY, Han, TY, Kim, IS, et al. "The Effects of 830 nm Light-Emitting Diode Therapy on Acute Herpes Zoster Ophthalmicus: A Pilot Study." *Annals of Dermatology.* 25(2):163–167, May 2013.

20. Fusco, BM, Giacovazzo, M. "Peppers and pain. The promise of capsaicin." *Drugs.* 53(6):909–914, June 1997.

21. Rice, ASC, et al. "EMA401, an orally administered highly selective angiotensin II type 2 receptor antagonist, as a novel treatment for postherpetic neuralgia: a randomized, double-blind, placebo-controlled phase 2 clinical trial." *The Lancet.* 1637–1647, May 2014.

22. De Luca, C, Kharaeva, Z, Raskovic, D, et al. "Coenzyme Q10, vitamin E, selenium, and methionine in the treatment of chronic recurrent viral mucocutaneous infections." *Nutrition.* 28(5):509–514, May 2012.

Chapter 2. Aging

1. Epel, ES, Blackburn, EH, Lin, J, et al. "Accelerated telomere shortening in response to life stress." *Proceedings of the National Academy of Science USA.* 101(49), 2004.

17312-5, http://www.ncbi.nlm.nih.gov/pubmed/15574496. Accessed November 6, 2013.

2. Robinson, MK, Tiesman, J, Binder, R, et al. "Immune and inflammatory gene expression profiles of chronological skin aging and photoaging." *Journal of the American Academy of Dermatology.* 58(2), 2008. AB_34, doi:10.1016/j.jaad.2007.10.163

3. Thornfeldt, CR. "Chronic inflammation is etiology of extrinsic aging." *Journal of Cosmetic Dermatology.* 7(1) 78–82, 2008. doi: 10.1111/j.1473-2165.2008.00366.x.

4. Putterman, E, Lin, J, Blackburn, E, et al. "The power of exercise: buffering the effect of chronic stress on telomere length." *PLoS One.* 5(5), 2010. e10837, doi: 10.1371/journal .pone.0010837. Accessed November 6, 2013.

5. Woolston, C. "Of Course You are Stressed. Just Look at Your Face." *Los Angeles Times,* April 27, 2013.

6. Thuerk, S. "Lack of sleep may speed up skin aging." *Dermatology Times.* September 24, 2013. http://dermatologytimes.modernmedicine.com/dermatology-times/news/lack-sleep-may-speed-skin-aging

7. Ornish, D, Lin, J, Chan, JM, et al. "Effect of comprehensive lifestyle changes on telomerase

activity and telomere length in men with biopsy-proven low-risk prostate cancer: 5-year follow-up of a descriptive pilot study." *Lancet Oncology.* (11):1112–1120. October 14, 2013.

8. Putterman, E, et al. 'The power of exercise: buffering the effect of chronic stress on telomere length." *PLoS One.* 5(5), 2010. e10837, doi: 10.1371/journal.pone.0010837. Accessed November 6, 2013.

9. Kellar, RS, Hubka, M, Rheins, LA, et al. "Hypoxic conditioned culture medium from fibroblasts grown under embryonic-like conditions supports healing following post-laser resurfacing." *Journal of Cosmetic Dermatology.* 8(3): 190–196, 2009. doi: 10.1111/j.1473-2165 .2009.00454.x.

10. Zimber, M. Mansbridge, J. Taylor, M, et al. "Human cell-conditioned media produced under embryonic-like conditions result in improved healing time after laser resurfacing." *Aesthetic Plastic Surgery.* 36 (2):43–437, 2012.

11. Laughlin, GA, Barrett-Connor, E. "Sexual Dimorphism in the Influence of Advanced Aging on Adrenal Hormone Levels: The Rancho Bernardo Study." *Journal of Clinical Endocrinoloigy and Metabolism.* 85 (10) 3561–3568, 2000.

12. Woods, NF, Mitchell, ES, Smith-DiJulio, K. "Cortisol Levels During the Menopausal Transition and Early Postmenopause: Observations from the Seattle Midlife Women's Health Study." *Menopause.* 16 (4): 708–718, 2009. doi: 10.1097/gme.0b013e318198d6b2.

13. Bitter, P, Pozner, J. "Retrospective Evaluation of the Long-term Antiaging Effects of BroadBand Light Therapy." *Cosmetic Dermatology.* 34–40, February 2013.

Chapter 3. Stress and Hair

1. Peters, EM, Liotiri, S, Bodó, E, et al. "Probing the effects of stress mediators on the human hair follicle: substance P holds central position." *American Journal of Pathology.* 171(6): 1872–1886, 2007. doi: 10.2353/ajpath.2007.061206

2. Ibid.

3. Arck, PC, Handjiski, B, Milena, E, et al. "Stress Inhibits Hair Growth in Mice by Induction of Premature Catagen Development and Deleterious Perifollicular Inflammatory Events via Neuropeptide Substance P-Dependent Pathways." *American Journal of Pathology.* 162(3) 803–814, 2003.

4. Hadshiew, IM, Foitzik, K, Arck, PC, et al. "Burden of hair loss: stress and the underestimated psychosocial impact of telogen effluvium and androgenetic alopecia." *The Journal of Investigative Dermatology.* 123(3):455–457, 2003.

5. Goosens, KA, Sapolsky, RM. "Stress and Glucocorticoid Contributions to Normal and Pathological Aging." in "Stress and Glucocorticoid Contributions to Normal and Pathological Aging." ed. DR Riddle, Boca Raton, FL": *CRC Press.* Ch 13, 2007.

6. Woods, NF, Mitchell, ES, Smith-DiJulio, K. "Cortisol Levels During the Menopausal Transition and Early Postmenopause Observations from the Seattle Midlife Women's Health Study." *Menopause.* 16(4): 708–718, 2009. doi: 10.1097/gme.0b013e318198d6b2.

Chapter 4. Nerves

1. Kendra, C. "The Peripheral Nervous System." netplaces.com. Accessed June 27, 2013. Last modified November 12, 2012.

2. Brody, J. "Scientists Cast Misery of Migraine in New Light." *The New York Times*. August 8, 2006.

3 American Accreditation HealthCare Commission, (A.D.A.M., Inc.—www.urac.org). "In Depth Report on Migraines: Causes." *The New York Times*. December 12, 2012.

4. Ibid

5. Sasannejad, P. Saeedi, M, Shoeibi, A, et al. "Lavender essential oil in the treatment of migraine headache: a placebo-controlled clinical trial." *European Neurology*. 67 (5):288–291, 2012. doi: 10.1159/000335249. Accessed November 25, 2013.

6. Vickers, AJ, Rees, RW, Zollman, CE, et al. "Acupuncture for chronic headache in primary care: large, pragmatic, randomized trial." *British Medical Journal*. 328(7442):744, 2004. doi: http://dx.doi.org/10.1136/bmj.38029.421863.

7. Mauskop, A. "Nonmedication, alternative, and complementary treatments for migraine," *Continuum (Minneap Minn)*. 18(4):796–806, 2012. doi: 10.1212/01.CON.0000418643.24408.40

8. Schellenberg, R. "Biofeedback in chronic headaches: at least as effective as drug therapy." *MMW Fortschritte De Medizin*. 154 (16):24, 2012.

9. Silberstein, S, Mathew, N, Saper, J, et al. "Botulinum toxin type A as a migraine preventive treatment." *Headache*. 40(6):445–450, 2000.

10. Greco, A, Gallo, A, Fusconi, M, et al. "Bell's palsy and autoimmunity." *Autoimmunity Reviews*. 12(2):323–328, 2012.

11. Gilden, DH. "Clinical practice. Bell's Palsy." *New England Journal of Medicine*. 351(13):1323–1331, 2004.

12. Sullivan, FM, et al. "Early treatment with prednisolone or acyclovir in Bell's palsy." *New England Journal of Medicine*. 357(16):1598–1607, 2007.

13. Kuga, M, Ikeda, M, Kukimoto, N, et al. "An assessment of physical and psychological stress of patients with facial paralysis." *Nihon Jibiinkoka Gakkai Kaiho*. (Japanese) 101(11) 1321–1327, 1998. Quoted in Huang, B, Xu, S, Xiong, J, et al."Psychological factors are closely associated with the Bell's palsy: A case-control study." *Journal of Huazhong University of Science and Technology* [*Medical Sciences*] 32(2):272–279, 2012.

14 Cumberworth, A. Mabvuure, NT, Norris, JM, et al. "Is acupuncture beneficial in the treatment of Bell's palsy?: best evidence topic (BET)." *International Journal of Surgery*. 10(6):310–312, 2012.

Chapter 5. Meditation

1. Bailey, NA. *Universal Etymological English Dictionary*. London: Columbia University, 1773.

2. Everly, GS, Lating, JM. *A Clinical Guide to the Treatment of Human Stress Response*. New York, NY: Springer, 2013.

3. Jacobs, TL, Epel, ES, Lin, J, et al. "Intensive meditation training, immune cell telomerase activity, and psychological mediators." *Psychoneuroendocrinology*. 36(5):664–681, 2011.

4. Dreher, D. *The Tao of Inner Peace*. New York, NY: First Plume Printing, 2000.

5. Yogananda, P. *Autobiography of a Yogi*. Crystal Clarity Publishers, Inc. Nevada City, CA: Reprint of the 1946 first edition, 2005.

6. Carlson, LE, Speca, M, Patel, KD, et al. "Mindfulness-based stress reduction in relation to quality of life, mood, symptoms of stress, and levels of cortisol, dehydroepiandrosterone sulfate (DHEAS) and melatonin in breast and prostate cancer outpatients." *Psychoneuroendocrinology*. 29(4):448–474, 2004.

7. Eppley, KR, Abrams, AI, Shear, J. "Differential effects of relaxation techniques on trait anxiety: a meta-analysis." *Journal of Clinical Psychology*. 45(6):957–974, 1989.

8. Bood, SA, Sundequist, U, Kjellgren, A, et al. "Effects of floatation-restricted environmental stimulation technique on stress-related muscle pain: what makes the difference in therapy—attention-placebo or the relaxation response?" *Pain Research and Management*. 10(4):201–209, 2005.

9. Schulz, P, Kaspar, CH "Neuroendocrine and psychological effects of restricted environmental stimulation technique in a floatation tank," *Biological Psychology*. 37(2):161–175, 1994.

Chapter 6. Massages

1. Field, T, Hernandez-Reif, M, Diego, M, et al. "Cortisol decreases and serotonin and dopamine increase following massage therapy." *International Journal of Neuroscience*. 115(10):1397–1413, 2005.

2. Moraska, A, Pollini, RA, Boulanger, K, et al. "Physiological adjustments to stress measures following massage therapy: a review of the literature." *Evidence-Based Complementary and Alternative Medicine*. 7(4):409–418, 2010.

Chapter 7. Breath and Movement

1. Huang, CJ, Webb, HE, Zourdos, MC, et al. "Cardiovascular reactivity, stress, and physical activity." *Frontiers in Physiology*. 4: 314, 2013.

2. Salmon, P. "Effects of physical exercise on anxiety, depression, and sensitivity to stress: a unifying theory." *Clinical Psychology Review*. 1.33–61, 2001.

http://www.ncbi.nlm.nih.gov/pubmed/11148895.

3. Schoenfeld, TJ, Rada, P, Pieruzzini, PR, et al. "Physical exercise prevents stress-induced activation of granule neurons and enhances local inhibitory mechanisms in the dentate gyrus." *Journal of Neuroscience*. 33(18):7770–7777, 2013. doi: 10.1523/JNEUROSCI.5352-12.2013.

4. Gopal, A, Mondal, S, Gandhi, A, et al. "Effect of integrated yoga practices on immune responses in examination stress-a preliminary study." *International Journal of Yoga*. 4(1):26–32, 2011. doi: 10.4103/0973-6131.78178.

5. Malathi, A, Damodaran, A. "Stress due to exams in medical students—role of yoga," *Indian Journal of Physiology and Pharmacology*. 43(2):218–224, 1999. http://www.ijpp.com/IJPP%20archives/1999_43_2/218-224.pdf.

Chapter 8. Acupuncture

1. Basser, S. "Acupuncture: A History." *Scientific Review Of Alternative Medicine*. 3:34–41, 1999.

2. Bonavita, B, Lo, Y. *First International Conference on the Physical, Chemical and Biological Properties of Stable Water Clusters*. Los Angeles, CA: World Science Publishing Co. 1977.

3. Ernst, E. White, AR, eds. *Acupuncture: A Scientific Appraisal*. Oxford: GB, Butterworth Heinemann, 1999.

4. *Acupuncture at ST36 prevents chronic stress-induced increases in neuropeptide Y in rat.* Eshkevari L, Egan R, Phillips D, Tilan J, Carney E, Azzam N, Amri H, Mulroney SE. *Exp Biol Med* (Maywood). 2012 Jan;237(1):18-23. doi: 10.1258/ebm.2011.011224. Epub 2011 Dec 7.

5. Mooney, T. "Diagnosis and management of patients with Bell's palsy," *Nursing Standard*. 28(14):44–49, 2013.

6. Fang, J, Zheng, N, Wang, Y, et al. "Understanding Acupuncture Based on ZHENG Classification from System Perspective." *Evidence-Based Complementary and Alternative Medicine*. 2013.

7. Wang, L, Zhao, B, Zhou, L. "Status and strategies analysis on international standardization of auricular acupuncture points." *Traditional Chinese Medicine*. 33(3):408–412, 2013):

8. Lao, L, Huang, L, Feng, C, et al. "Evaluating traditional Chinese medicine using modern clinical trial design and statistical methodology: application to a randomized controlled acupuncture trial." *Statistics in Medicine*. 31(7):619–627, 2012.

9. Kalauokalani, D, Cherkin, DC, Sherman, KJ. "A comparison of physician and nonphysician acupuncture treatment for chronic low back pain," The *Clinical Journal of Pain*. 21(5):406–411, 2005.

10. Shin, KR, Ha, JY, Park HJ, et al. "The effect of hand acupuncture therapy and hand moxibustion therapy on premenstrual syndrome among Korean women." *Western Journal of Nursing Research*. 31(2):171–186, 2009.

11. Mayo Clinic. "Acupuncture And Myofascial Trigger Therapy Treat Same Pain Areas." *ScienceDaily*. www.sciencedaily.com/releases/2008/05/080513101614.htm. Accessed January 28, 2014.

12. Sun, PS, et al. "The study on conduction of acoustic information along meridians." *Chen Tzu Yen Chiu* 13(2):139–143, 1988.

13. Shin, W. "The effect of convalescent meridian acupressure after exercise on stress hormones and lactic acid concentration changes." *Journal of Exercise Rehabilitation*. 9(2):331–335, 2013.

Chapter 9. Diet and Supplements

1. Huynh, M, Gupta, R, and Yoo, JYM. "Emotional Stress as a Trigger for Inflammatory Skin Disorders." *Seminars in Cutaneous Medicine and Surgery.* 32:68–72, 2013.

2. Chilton, F, Tucker, L. *Win the War Within: The Eating Plan That's Clinically Proven to Fight Inflammation—The Hidden Cause of Weight Gain and Chronic Disease.* New York, NY: Simon & Schuster, 2006.

3. Ibid.

4. Perricone, N. *The Perricone Promise: Look Younger Live Longer in Three Easy Steps.* New York, NY: Warner Brothers, 2004.

5. Ibid.

6. Ibid.

7. Soni, S, Badawy, SZ. "Celiac disease and its effect on human reproduction: a review," *Journal of Reproductive Medicine.* 55 1–2, 3–8, 2010.

8. Credicott, T. *The Healthy Gluten-Free Life: 200 Delicious Gluten-Free, Dairy-Free, Soy-Free, and Egg-Free Recipes.* Riverside, NJ: Victory Belt Publishing, a Simon & Schuster imprint, 2013.

9. Murray, M. *The Pill Book Guide to Natural Medicines.* New York, NY: Bantam Books, 2002.

10. Murzaku, EC, Bronsnick, T, Rao, BK. "Diet in Dermatology: Part II. Melanoma, chronic urticaria, and psoriasis." *Journal of the American Academy of Dermatology.* 1053–1064, December 2014.

11. Nguyen, TA, Friedman, AJ. "Curcumin: A Novel Treatment for Skin-Related Disorders. *Journal of Drugs in Dermatology.* 12(10): 1131–1137, October 2013.

12. Choudhry, SZ, Bhatia, N Ceilley, R, et al. "Role of Oral Polypodium Leucotomos Extract in Dermatologic Diseases: A Review of the Literature." *Journal of Drugs in Dermatology.* 13(2): 148–153, February 2014.

13. Fomichev, VI, Pchelintsev, VP. "The Neurohumoral systems of patients with ischemic heart disease and under emotional pain stress: the means for their pharmacologic regulation." Kardiologlia. 33(10):15–18, 1993.

14. Kambayashi H, Odake Y, Takada K, et al. "N-retinoyl-D-glucosamine, a new retinoic acid agonist, mediates topical retinoid efficacy with no irritation on photoaged skin." *British Journal of Dermatology.* 153(Suppl2):30–36, 2005.

15. Bissett, DL. "Glucosamine: an ingredient with skin and other benefits. *Journal of Cosmetic Dermatology.* 5:309–315, 2006.

16. Banderet, LE, Lieberman, HR. "Treatment with tyrosine, a neurotransmitter precursor, reduces environmental stress in humans." *Brain Research Bulletin.* 22(4):759–762, 1989.

17. Bronsnick, T, Murzaku, EC, Rao, BK. "Diet in Dermatology:Part I :Atopic dermatitis, acne, and nonmelanoma skin cancer. *Journal of the American Academy of Dermatology.* 1039–1050, December 2014.

18. Ibid.

19. Ablon, G. "A Double-Blind Placebo-Controlled Study Evaluating the Efficacy of an Oral Supplement." *Journal of Clinical and Aesthetic Dermatology*. 5(11): 28–34, November 2012.

Chapter 10. Psychotherapy

1. Huynh, H, Gupta, R, Koo, JY. "Emotional stress as a trigger for inflammatory skin disorders." *Seminars in Cutaneous Medicine and Surgery*. 32(2):68–72, 2013. Review.

2. Cushman, P. *Constructing The Self, Constructing America: A Cultural History Of Psychotherapy*. Boston, MA: Da Capo Press, 1996.

3. Norcross, JC, Vandenbos, GR, Freedheim, DK. *History of Psychotherapy: Continuity and Change*. American Psychological Assoc. Washington, DC, 2011.

4. Markowitz, JC, Weissman, MM. "Interpersonal psychotherapy: principles and applications," *World Psychiatry* 3(3):136–139, 2004.

5. Ibid.

6. Welfare-Wilson, A, Newman, R. "Cognitive behavioural therapy for psychosis and anxiety." *British Journal of Nursing*. 22(18):1061–1065, 2013.

7. Parrish, BP, Cohen, LH, Gunthert, KC, et al. "Effects of Cognitive Therapy for Depression on Daily Stress-Related Variables." *Behavior Research and Therapy*. 47(5): 444–448, 2009.

doi: 10.1016/j.brat.2009.02.005

8. Huynh, M, Gupta, R, Koo, JY. "Emotional stress as a trigger for inflammatory skin disorders." *Seminars in Cutaneous Medicine and Surgery*. 32(2):68–72, 2013. Review.

9. Schneider, KJ, Langle, A. "The renewal of humanism in psychotherapy: summary and conclusion." *Psychotherapy (Chic)*. 49(4):480–481, 2012.

doi: 10.1037/a0028026.

10. Barsaglini, A, Sartori, G, Benetti, S, et al. "The effects of psychotherapy on brain function: A systematic and critical review." *Progress in Neurobiology*. 2013.

doi: 10.1016/j.pneurobio.2013.10.006.

Chapter 11. Light-Emitting Diodes

1. Whelan, HT, Smits, RL, et al. "Effect of NASA Light-Emitting Diode Irradiation on Wound Healing. "*Journal of Clinical Laser Medicine Surgery*, 19(6), 2004. http://online.liebertpub.com/doi/abs/10.1089/104454701753342758. Accessed June 17, 2013.

2. Griffin, S. "LED Lights Skin Care." Livestrong. www.livestrong.com Last modified October 13, 2010. Accessed June 17, 2013.

3. Whelan, HT, Smits, RL, et al. "Effect of NASA Light-Emitting Diode Irradiation on Wound Healing." *Journal of Clinical Laser Medicine Surgery*. 19(6), 2004.

4. Lev-Tov, H, Mamalis, A, Brody, N, et al. "Inhibition of Fibroblast Proliferation In Vitro Using Red Light-Emitting Diodes." *Dermatologic Surgery*. 39:1167–1170, 2013.

5. Alcantara, CC, Gigo-Benato, D, Salvini, TF, et al. "Effect of Low-Level Laser Therapy (LLLT) on Acute Neural Recovery and Inflammation-Related Gene Expression After Crush Injury in Rat Sciatic Nerve." *Lasers in Surgery and Medicine.* 45:246–252, 2013.

6. Lanzafame, RJ, Blanche, RR, Bodian, AB, et al. "The growth of human scalp hair mediated by visible red light laser and LED sources in males." *Lasers in Surgery and Medicine.* 45:487–495, 2013.

7. Avcu, P, Gupta, A, Sadasivam, M, et al. "Low-Level Laser (Light) Therapy (LLLT) in Skin: Stimulating, Healing, Restoring." *Seminars in Cutaneous Medicine and Surgery* 32:41–52, 2013.

8. Ablon, G. "Combination 830-nm and 633-nm Light-Emitting Diode Phototherapy Shows Promise in the Treatment of Recalcitrant Psoriasis: Preliminary Findings." *Photomedicine and Laser Surgery.* 28(2): 141–146, 2010.

Chapter 12. Electrical Stimulation

1. Rohde, C, Chiang, A, Adipoju, O, et al. "Effects of Pulsed Electromagnetic Fields on IL-1B amd Post Operative Pain: A Double-Blind, Placebo-Controlled Pilot Study in Breast Reduction Patients." *Plastic and Reconstructive Surgery* 125(6):1620–1629, 2010.

2. Strauch, B, Herman, C, Dabb, R, et al. "Evidence-Based Use of Pulsed Electromagnetic Therapy in Clinical Plastic Surgery." *Aesthetic Surgery Journal* 29(2):135–143, 2009.

3. Allen, JK, Blanchard, EB. "Biofeedback-based stress management training with a population of business managers." *Biofeedback and Self Regulation.* 5(4):427–438, 1980.

4. Sutarto, AP, Wahab, MN, Zin, NM. "Resonant breathing biofeedback training for stress reduction among manufacturing operators." *International Journal of Occupational Safety and Ergonomics.* 18(4):549–561, 2012.

Chapter 13. Over-The-Counter Products and Prescription Medications

1. Kannan, S, Lim, HW. "Photoprotection and Vitamin D: A review. Photodermatology Photoimmunology Photomedicine." http://dx.doi.org/10.1111/phpp.12096. January 9 2014.

2. Chen, L, Hu, JY, Wang, SQ. "The role of antioxidants in photoprotection: a critical review." *Journal of the American Academy of Dermatology.* 67(5): 1013–1024, November 2012.

doi: 10.1016/j.jaad.2012.02.009.

3. Farris, P, Krutmann, J, Yan-Hong, L, et al. "Reservatrol: A Unique Antioxidant Offering a Multi-Mechanistic Approach for Treating Aging Skin." *Journal of Drugs in Dermatology.* 12(12):1389-1394, December 2013.

4. Ferzli, G, Patel, M, Phrsai, N, et al. "Reduction of Facial Redness with Resveratrol Added to Topical Product Containing Green Tea Poyphenols and Caffeine." *Journal of Drugs in Dermatology.* 12 (7): 770–774, July 2013.

5. Boyd, A. "The Role for Resveratrol in the Skin Care Regimen." *Modern Aesthetics.*: 58–59, March 2014.

6. Shytle, DR, Tan, J, Ehrhart, J, et al. "Effects of blue-green algae extracts on the proliferation of human adult stem cells in vitro: a preliminary study." *Medical Science Monitor.* 16(1)::BR1-5, January 2010.

7. Pirot, F, Millet, J, Kalia, YN, et al. "In vitro study of percutaneous absorption, cutaneous bioavailability and bioequivalence of zinc and copper from five topical formulations." *Skin Pharmacology.* 9:259–269, 1996.

8. Maggini, S, Wintergerst, ES, Beveridge, S, et al. "Selected vitamins and trace elements support immune function by strengthening epithelial barriers and cellular and humoral immune responses." *British Journal of Nutrition.* 98(Suppl 1): S29–35. Review. October 2007.

9 Lupo, MP, Cole, AL."Cosmeceutical Peptides." *Dermatology Therapy.* 20(5):343–349, 2007.

10. Kornhauser, A, Wei, RR, Yamaguchi, Y, et al. "The effects of topically applied glycolic acid and salicylic acid on ultraviolet radiation-induced erythema, DNA damage and sunburn cell formation in human skin." *Journal of Dermatological Science.* 55(1):10–17 July2009.

11. Draelos, ZD. "Modern moisturizer myths, misconceptions, and truths." *Cutis.* 91(6): 308–314, June 2013.

12. Briganti, S, Camera, E, Picardo, M. "Chemical and instrumental approaches to treat hyperpigmentation." *Pigment Cell Research.* 16:1–11. 2003.

13. Shankaran, V. Brooks, M, Mostow, E. "Advanced therapies for chronic wounds: NPWT, engineered skin, growth factors, extracellular matrices." *Dermatology Therapy.* 26(3):215–221, May-June 2013.

14. Kellar, RS, Hubka, M, Rheins, LA, et al. "Hypoxic conditioned culture medium from fibroblasts grown under embryonic-like conditions supports healing following post-laser resurfacing." *Journal of Cosmetic Dermatology.* 8(3):190–196, 2009.

15. Zimber, MP, Mansbridge, JN, Taylor, M et al. "Human cell-conditioned media produced under embryonic-like conditions result in improved healing time after laser resurfacing." *Aesthetic Plastic Surgery.* 36(2):431–437, 2012.

16. "Studies Highlight Potential Breakthrough in Embryonic Stem Cells Production." *Dermatology Daily.* Thursday, January 30, 2014. http://aad.bulletinhealthcare.com.

17. Draelos, ZD. "Glycobiology and the Skin: A New Frontier." *A Supplement to Cutis.* 8–10, February 2013.

18. Rawlings, AV, Boegeli, R. "Stratum Corneum Proteases and Dry Skin Condtitions." *Cell and Tissue Research.* 351(2): 217–235. October 9, 2012.

doi: 10.1007/s00441-012-1501-x.

19. Putterman, E, Lin, J, Blackburn, E, et al. "The power of exercise: buffering the effect of chronic stress on telomere length." *PLoS One.* 5(5), 2010.

20. Epel, EDS, Blackburn, EH, Lin, J, et al. "Accelerated telomere shortening in response to life stress." *Proceedings of the National Academy of Sciences of the United States of America.* 101(49):17312–17315, 2004.

21. Epel, E,. Daubenmier, J, Moskowitz, JT, el al. "Can meditation slow rate of cellular aging? Cognitive stress, mindfulness and telomeres." *Annals of New York Academy of Sciences.* 1172 34–53, 2009.

22. Draelos, ZD. *Cosmeceuticals.* (Philadelphia, PA: Elsevier, 2005.

23. Wolf, R. Parish, LC. "Barrier-repair prescription moisturizers: do we really need them? Facts and controversies." *Clinics in Dermatology.* 31(6):787–791, November-December 2013.

21. Del Rosso, J, Cash, K. "Topical Corticosteroid Application and the Structural and Functional Integrity of the Epidermal Barrier." *The Journal of Clinical and Aesthetic Dermatology.* 6(111):20–26. November 2013.

24. Prussick, L, Prussick, R. "Vitamin D and Psoriasis." *Practical Dermatology.* 27–28. November 2013.

25. Ablon, G. "A Double-Blind Placebo-Controlled Study Evaluating the Efficacy of an Oral Supplement." *Journal of Clinical and Aesthetic Dermatology.* 5(11): 28–34. November 2012.

Chapter 14. Non-Invasive Procedures

1. Bitter, P, Pozner, J. "Retrospective Evaluation of the Long-term Antiaging Effects of Broad-Band Light Therapy." *Cosmetic Dermatology.* 34–40. February 2013.

2. Smith, SR, Jones, D, Thomas, JA, Murphy, DK, et al. "Duration of wrinkle correction following repeat treatment with Juvéderm hyaluronic acid fillers." *Archhives of Dermatological Research.* 302(10):757–762. December 2010.

3. R Jandhyala, "Impact of botulinum toxin a on the quality of life of subjects following treatment of facial lines," *Journal of Clinical Aesthetic Dermatology.* 6(9):41–45. September 2013.

4. Alam, M, Barrett, KC, Hodapp, RM, et al. "Botulinum toxin and the facial feedback hypotheses:can looking better make you feel happier?" *Journal of the American Academy of Dermatology.* 58(6):1061–1072. June 2008.

5. Koch, D. Pratsou, P, Szczecinska, W, et al. "The diverse application of laser hair removal therapy: a tertiary laser unit's experience with less common indications and a literature overview." *Lasers in Medical Science.* Oct 31, 2013. [Epub ahead of print].

6. Chung, H, Dai, T, Sharma, SK, et al. "The nuts and bolts of low-level laser (light) therapy." *Annals of Biomedical Engineering.* 40(2): 516–533. February 2012.

7. J Chen, Y Qiu, S Zhang, G Yang, Y Gao. "Controllable coating of microneedles for transdermal drug delivery." *Drug Development and Industrial Pharmacy.* (Epub ahead of print). December 2013.

Index

About the Authors

Glynis Ablon, M.D., F.A.A.D.

Dr. Ablon is an acclaimed dermatologist, cosmetic surgeon, and Associate Clinical Professor of Dermatology at UCLA who runs a thriving practice in the Los Angeles area. Dr. Ablon subscribes to the philosophy that, in order to treat the issues of the skin, she has to treat the whole person, and is known for her holistic approach with her patients. As founder of the Ablon Skin Institute and Research Center, she guides pioneering research in dermatology products and procedures. She has frequently been called upon to share her knowledge as an on-camera medical consultant for such shows as *The Talk, The Doctors, Entertainment Tonight,* and *Extra Television,* and has appeared on such networks as: ABC, CBS, E! Entertainment, Lifetime, Oxygen, Fox Television, and Canadian Television.

Dr. Ablon studied dermatology at George Washington University Medical School in the District of Columbia, and completed her residency training in dermatology at Baylor College of Medicine in Houston, Texas. Early on, she focused on cosmetic surgery and performed a fellowship in oculoplastic surgery at the Sinskey Eye Institute in Santa Monica, California. Dr. Ablon's cosmetic certification extends from injectable fillers and toxins to laser surgery, liposuction, blepharoplasty, and sclerotherapy.

In addition to practicing medicine, Dr. Ablon has published a large body of research and has presented her work at multiple medical symposiums and conferences, including the prestigious International Master Course on Aging Skin (IMCAS) in Paris, France. Her drive to discover innovative approaches to dermatology led her to found the Ablon Skin Institute (ASI) Research Center, which serves as an independent clinical research site specializing in dermatologic clinical trials. The center, with its full-time research staff, has over sixteen years of research experience. It has worked closely with the Western Institutional Review Board, and has an excellent reputation for presenting accurate data.

Dr. Ablon is a fellow of the American Academy of Dermatology, American Academy of Liposuction Surgery, American Society for Laser Medicine and Surgery, American Society for Dermatologic Surgery, Women's Dermatologic Surgery, and the Skin Cancer Foundation, to name a few.

Susanna DeSimone, M.F.A.

Ms. DeSimone graduated Magna Cum Laude from University of California, Berkeley, then went on to earn a Master of Fine Arts from Loyola Marymount University. As a writer, she pairs with experts in the fields of health and self-help to craft informative non-fiction works. She also teaches at the university level. For more details about this author and her works, please refer to DesignerBooks.org.